CW01263811

Why Bipolar?

The Demystification of
Bipolar Affective Disorder

Declan Henry

Copyright © Declan Henry 2013

First published by Squirrel Publishing 2013

Reprinted 2017

A CIP catalogue record for this book is available from the British Library.

ISBN 978-0-9576893-0-5

Prepared and printed by:

York Publishing Services Ltd
64 Hallfield Road
Layerthorpe
York YO31 7ZQ

Tel: 01904 431213

Website: www.yps-publishing.co.uk

This book is dedicated to the youth of the future that they will grow up to live in a world free of psychiatry and the misuse of psychotropic drugs.

Going to a psychiatrist has become one of the most dangerous things a person can do.

Peter Breggin, MD

Disclaimer to Life Stories

The 26 life stories contained in this book were collected from a random selection of men and women with bipolar in Ireland and the UK, who willingly responded to my request to hear their stories. The people featured came from different age groups, backgrounds, socio-economic standings, sexual orientations and religious beliefs. Amongst those who participated there were various levels of insight, although many were highly knowledgeable of their condition. (Naturally, names and some other details have been changed to protect identities and anonymity.)

Preface

Lady Margaret McNair

President

Citizens Commission on Human Rights UK

There is no doubt that life can be described in many varied ways; it can be fun, exhilarating, enjoyable, challenging, demanding, taxing, stressful, disappointing, overwhelming, insurmountable, even impossible. The list of adjectives can go on and on, changing along with the viewpoint of the person giving the answers.

Of course, people view life in different ways from their own unique perspectives, with their own idiosyncratic thoughts on life, the universe and everything. From an insurmountable, impossible, untenable position, to a fun exhilarating existence, we all have our own unique stories to tell of how we made it through the hard times, how we survived what life threw at us, all the way up to the dizzy heights of how we achieved success in the face of adversity, how we overcame barriers to achieve the goals we set ourselves, goals we thought we would never see come to fruition.

So it is that we weather the troughs and ride the crests of each day, making what we hope will be the right decisions as we confront the ups and downs that constitute everyday living.

For some however, those troughs and crests take on greater meaning when their lives are inadvertently moulded by the extremes that are described in psychiatric circles as manic, extreme highs and extreme lows, and which have been unscientifically labelled by the psychiatric fraternity as so-called 'bipolar disorder'.

Formerly known as manic depression, bipolar disorder is the label given to those who hit the depths of despair one day, while experiencing the exultation and euphoria of a job well done the next. But, I hear you ask, isn't that normal? Isn't it a regular feature to go up and down in life? One could say, "Welcome to planet Earth." But this particular see-saw of emotions is as different from the normal ups and downs of life as a tsunami is from a swimming pool. Hell's see-saw of extremes remains as debilitating today as it was decades or even centuries ago. It is not a new concept – unless you're in the psychiatric business looking for new ideas.

After all, the title *bipolar disorder* makes it sound as though it hails from an educated fraternity that has complete empathy and understanding for the emotional extremes that blight individual lives. In reality however, that is not the case. It is an invented mental illness that has already changed its name once – manic depression aka bipolar disorder. You or I could take a human behaviour of which we disapprove or upon which we frown, and redefine it. For example, in the 19th century, women were described as having nervous hysteria – which sounds equally knowledgeable and official, like an ailment for which there is a cure. Most, it turns out, were merely socially and sexually frustrated by the strictures of the society in which they lived.

Well-funded psychiatric studies rely heavily on the use of weasel words to hoodwink the public into believing something sensible is being said when a particular type of behaviour is magnified. The Oxford Dictionary describes a weasel word as "an equivocal or ambiguous word used intentionally to mislead". It is a fitting term for psychiatry in general because well-funded psychiatric studies and drug literature rely heavily on the use of these words.

Using weasel words, pharmaceutical companies describe their products as treating the symptoms of bipolar disorder, claiming the condition to be *probably* caused by a chemical imbalance in the brain. You get the impression something meaningful is being said, when in fact they are vague or meaningless claims.

Highly-paid laboratory technicians come up with new recipes that are marketed as magic bullets to guide a person through the dark times that go hand-in-hand with bipolar. At which point, the stage is set. Cue the drum roll and enter the apparent saviours; the psycho-pharmaceutical liberators of mental suffering, otherwise known as psychiatrists, working alongside and perpetuating an unholy alliance with Big Pharma, otherwise known as the pharmaceutical industry or just plain old drug companies – pushers in very nice suits.

In reality however, what they have done is to concoct an expensive chemical crutch that generates a debilitating sensation, putting the person in a chemical haze, a haze which is then described as demonstrably effective, on the spurious basis that a haze is better than a depression. All that has actually happened is the person has been drugged and is demonstrating the effects of having taken a substance that has caused him or her to malfunction when the natural chemical processes of the body are disturbed.

While bipolar disorder is entirely *unscientific*, it is being pushed, promoted and promulgated along with other psychiatric labels, ensconced in even more weasel words to give it that scientific credibility to make it into the condition that will reap the sought-after financial rewards. To put it bluntly, shareholders expect to see a return on their investment. So if you're a psychiatrist with vested interests or a shareholder in a pharmaceutical company that has just developed the new blockbuster drug for bipolar, the ups and downs in life have never been so good! An investigation, prompted by Senator Charles Grassely, was conducted by Harvard University-affiliated Massachusetts General Hospital. In July 2011, it concluded that psychiatrist Joseph Biederman and two of his protégés, Thomas Spencer and Timothy Wilens – each of who failed to disclose millions of dollars they had each received from the makers of antipsychotics, the drugs they promoted for the treatment of bipolar in children – had violated the University's and hospital's conflict of interest reporting standards (1).

This marketing strategy for bipolar, as well as other psychiatric labels, is helping to bring about what is being described as a mental health monopoly, a situation where psychiatric interventions are accepted as the answer to virtually all of life's perceived problems. The contemporary habit of prescribing antidepressants for premenstrual syndrome is an example. Such a marketing strategy is reliant of course upon the ignorance of you and I and people in general.

So the mental health monopoly is covertly established, continuing to gain credibility through the cultivation of conditions like bipolar where their medical status can be elevated to a plateau where they sit alongside real, validated diseases.

We can see the promulgation of conditions like bipolar by virtue of their use in everyday language. 'Bipolar' this, 'bipolar' that, "I'm having a bipolar day", "My cat has bipolar", the term has entered our language as an adjective to describe the ups and downs in life or to simply label the motion, giving it more unwarranted credibility, thus strengthening its presence in society.

If you and I knew the scientific void that exists across the psychiatric spectrum, in psychiatric evaluations, psychiatric studies, psychiatric diagnoses, in psychiatry in general, it would be acceptable and we would be entirely correct to place the subject in the genre of fiction, perhaps fantasy. Psychiatric texts could be found in the same genre as J K Rowling's *Harry Potter* or Terry Pratchett's *Discworld*, where one of the titles occasionally gets taken off of the shelf for a little late night escapism. It is a work of opinions, personal thoughts about behaviour patterns, etc. It is therefore written in the same way that a fictional author would convey his message: made up as he goes along, with no scientific basis, other than what is called for to make the story believable.

But no, the mental health industry is deadly serious, forging a monopoly through the redefinition of behaviours as mental illnesses, while calling on the Government for more and more appropriations to deal with the escalating problem of more and more mental ill-health, an escalation that is pushed, promoted and promulgated by – you guessed it – the psychiatric industry. Whichever way you look at it, that is exceptionally good business acumen, but extremely bad medicine, since it builds profit on the basis of potentially increasing, or at least maintaining, the suffering of patients. This scenario is however currently being accepted as fact.

Whatever political agenda are being practiced in a country at any given time, the Government is not likely to consider investment in an industry that is failing. That however *is* what is happening when it comes to mental health. The psychiatric industry continues to advertise its failures, not its successes, to gain more taxpayers' funds. Furthermore, the same industry promotes that more and more people are suffering mental illness. With investment levels in mental health in a new echelon, the benefactor, that's you and me, should expect results, but they are not forthcoming. Perhaps there is a factor at work, a factor that is extremely hard to confront, a factor that is hard to conceive in light of the Hippocratic Oath, but which is nevertheless present. That factor is encompassed in this rather bold statement: if psychiatry ever cured anyone, it would go out of business.

Such a statement segues smoothly into the Achilles Heel of the mental health monopoly. Unlike real doctors who practice real medicine, psychiatrists openly admit they are unable to cure their patients. If that were not startling enough, add on the fact that the cornerstone of psychiatry's disease model today is the theory that a brain-based, chemical imbalance causes mental illness.

Do a cursory Google search of electronic texts using the search terms 'chemical imbalance of the brain' and 'bipolar disorder' and you get pages of results that have these two terms joined at the hip. The results will tell you 'bipolar' is "...caused by a chemical imbalance in the brain" (2), "that bipolar is widely believed to be the result of chemical imbalances in the brain" (3), "...the chemical imbalance of the brain, associated with bipolar disorder..." (4) and so on. But also consider that psychiatrists, by their own admission, do not have a single scientific test to support or validate the existence of the so-called chemical imbalance. Diabetes on the other hand, is a biochemical imbalance. The definitive test for its presence is a high blood sugar balance level. The late Dr Thomas Szasz, Emeritus Professor of Psychiatry, summed it up in these words, "There is no blood or other biological test to ascertain the presence or absence of a mental illness, as there is for most bodily diseases. If such a test were developed (for what theretofore, had been considered a psychiatric illness), then the condition would cease to be a mental illness, and would be classified, instead, as a symptom of a bodily disease" (5).

In view of the fact that a 'chemical imbalance of the brain' has never been scientifically validated, the words of former President of the World Psychiatric Association, Norman Sartorius, have even greater meaning. He said, "The time when psychiatrists considered they could cure the mentally ill is gone. In the future, the mentally ill have to learn to live with their illness."

It thus comes down again to that psychiatric marketing strategy which has been pushing, promoting and multiplying at an alarming rate, relying on the man in the street to maintain his lemming attitude and blindly accept the false psychiatric information. It has been cleverly orchestrated by means of two dominating psychiatric texts, the *Diagnostic and Statistical Manual of Mental Disorders* (DSM), published by the American Psychiatric Association, and the *International Classification of Diseases and Related Health Problems – Mental Disorders Section* (ICD) published by the World Health Organization.

It is the 21st century marketing of madness, where invented disorders satisfy the profit-driven industry. While attempting to be scientific and highly esoteric, the psychiatric labelling process has also become the butt of jokes, where everyday habits have been redefined as mental illness, and where even today's habitual processes are under psychiatric scrutiny. Internet addiction has been conceived as a mental illness inciting various comical retorts. Binge eating disorder and hoarding disorder are also examples. We could all get inventive, open up our imaginations, and offer up even more possibilities.

Joking aside, these diagnostic texts are the Emperors' new suits. It is a simple task to listen to a person and match his or her description of their difficulties to a convenient label that lists those very difficulties. It is also easy to marry up the disorder to a list of recommended drugs, and fill out a prescription for those drugs.

Another aspect of psychiatric labelling that deserves mention, if only for its sheer nerve and marketing genius, is the aspect of NOS. We may be in a technological age but, in this instance, NOS does not stand for Network Operating System. It stands for Not Otherwise Specified, used when the mental disorder appears to fall within the larger category but does not meet the criteria of any specific disorder within that category. It is a category that makes diagnosing someone with a mental disorder a whole lot easier. Just when you thought you didn't fit one of the psychiatric pigeon holes, when you thought you might escape the labelling clutches of the psychiatric industry, along comes NOS. The acronym has been tagged onto a number of so-called disorders. For example, there is eating disorder NOS, personality disorder NOS, depressive disorder NOS, cognitive disorder NOS, anxiety disorder NOS, and yes, bipolar disorder NOS is also there, brazenly described as a catch-all category, that is "... diagnosed when the disorder does not fall within a specific subtype."

Consider again the viewpoint of a psychiatrist with vested interests or the viewpoint of a shareholder in a pharmaceutical company that is developing new drugs. Not Otherwise Specified generates the potential of a spectrum for bipolar or any other so-called disorder, a spectrum that can have a considerable number of gradations, but which at the end of the day, has profit written all over it. The diagnostic possibilities are immense, as are the drug prescriptions, as are the shareholder dividends.

The common denominator with any monopoly is the intention to corner the market, to gain exclusive control over a commercial activity. In consideration of bipolar in particular, it was worth looking to see if there was any other avenue that had been left untapped that could be pursued to maximise profits. What about childhood? Take a look at their behaviour: children have good days, they have bad days, they have the terrible-twos, they have screaming episodes and days or even weeks when they go up and down like yo-yos. Since there is no scientific basis for any mental disorder, it comes down to the opinion of a psychiatrist as to how this behaviour is interpreted. Take the permutations and combinations of various behaviour patterns, throw in some psychiatric rhetoric and some weasel words and yes, childhood bipolar disorder is invented. As if that wasn't stretching the boundaries, could it go any further? Well, yes. When observing an adult losing his or her temper, the unruly display is often described by the saying "spitting his dummy out", or "throwing his toys out of the pram". Bearing these in mind, consider this: a new temper tantrum disorder is being considered to diagnose large numbers of children whose tantrums don't yet qualify them for bipolar disorder. The new diagnosis 'Temper Dysregulation with Dysphoria Disorder' broadens the bipolar disorder into a whole new category for children 0–3 years old. And the monopoly is complete.

Just as it is that we follow the doctor's recommendations, so it is that this labelling charade is proliferated through the trust placed in the authoritative personnel, the psychiatrist. When the house is on fire, we are confident the fire brigade will arrive to put it out. We welcome the firemen in without question to sort out the problem. When there is an accident on the motorway, we are confident the police and ambulance service will be alerted to come to the rescue, and we are pleased to see the blue flashing lights approaching. These are public institutions that provide a valuable service in times of need where the results are the all important factor.

It would be an immense pleasure to put psychiatry in this same category, but it simply doesn't meet the standards.

What percentage of people would be truly pleased to see the psychiatrist walking up the garden path with a crisis team in tow? What percentage of psychiatric treatments has a positive outcome? What percentage of people experiencing a personal crisis would really want to be involuntarily locked up with others who are having similar crises?

Another element strengthening the mental health monopoly and which separates psychiatry from all other fields in medicine is forced, involuntary treatment. The powers bestowed upon psychiatrists in the application of the Mental Health Act 1983 allow for involuntary detention, where a person can be locked up without having committed a crime, and where the person can be treated against his or her will, where dangerous, mind-altering drugs can be given without consent.

Those diagnosed with bipolar may have experienced the psychiatric enforcement procedures, where civil liberties are severely reduced if not completely erased in an instant, and where a drugged stupor can be instilled through forced treatment. There is no doubt that psychiatrists will have worked out in their own minds how to justify these punitive measures, so that they can sleep at night. It is a factor however that puts it in a brand new branch of medicine: punitive medicine. In any other specialty such as cardiology, geriatrics or oncology, the patient has a choice of whether to go ahead with any proposed treatment. They are allowed to exercise their fundamental human right of making a fully informed choice and thus give informed consent on whether or not they choose to go ahead. In psychiatry, this right can be stripped away through the application of mental health laws, giving it a unique yet notorious status in the medical field.

Addressing bipolar would not be complete without mentioning the psychiatric medications that are routinely prescribed. Hardly anyone had heard of the term mood stabiliser in 1995 when a license was granted to use the anticonvulsant sodium valproate to treat 'acute mania'. But today, the term 'mood stabiliser' is well known. It would be easy to be fooled by the argument that the advent of these classifications of drugs has replaced the psychiatric brutality of yesteryear. One of the main drugs prescribed for mood disorders is Lithium, a mineral given in salt form. It is a substance that can be extremely dangerous, since in order to achieve a 'sedating' effect, the 'therapeutic' dosage psychiatrists must use is so poisonous that it can cause serious harm or even death. What is worse, the body does not break down and metabolise Lithium very well. To remove it from the body, the kidneys are put under great stress to eliminate through urination. According to experts, the almost inevitable result of extensive Lithium use is kidney damage.

It is even more hazardous when too much of it accumulates in the body. Prolonged exposure to Lithium can lead to permanent brain damage and death. So much for the sound, humane, contemporary approach.

All that has happened is the brutality is now easier to witness. There is still no basis for mental illness. Anyone of sound mind would argue that to solve a problem, the problem must first be understood. In real medicine for example, if a doctor was preparing to remove a problematic tumour, he would need to understand what a tumour was and how it was troubling the patient. Anything else would be guessing, a term that is the height of blasphemy in scientific circles. It is worth returning to the idea of the elusive 'chemical imbalance'. Psychiatrists tell their patients that it is this that is at the root of their problem, although they know that no scientific test exists to validate this concept.

The conclusion is that we are witnessing a swindle unlike any that has gone before it, a swindle that extends into research establishments in universities and other organisations around the world. Let's not be shy about coming forward here: Big Pharma funds are extensive, and can be used to bring about favourable outcomes for their products. The Influence of the Pharmaceutical Industry covered this in a 2005 report. It said the industry spends £1.65 billion a year on marketing and promotional efforts while the Department of Health spends £4.5 million. It went further, stating: "In addition to receiving visits from company representatives, doctors are invited to attend sponsored events, meetings, workshops and symposia, which may be little more than 'hospitality masquerading as education'."

By monopolising this route, inexpensive non-drug solutions are met with a dull thud of the drum rather than the same fanfare. In fact, rarely do they get off the ground, due to a lack of research funding. If the non-drug solution should make it through the research phase, the mental health monopoly simply kicks in again when medical journals refuse to publish the research findings.

Big Pharma funds meant the all-important monopoly could be established far more rapidly. As well as the ignorance of the man in the street, which was and continues to be priceless, the pharmaceutical funds could also buy the advertising space, it could buy the research results, it could buy the alliances with those in high places or the favourable word to get that remunerative contract. Like the board game *Monopoly*, the winner is the one who purchases the most property, the one who has the most financial clout, the one who buys his way to the top. As in the board game, the real life monopoly in the mental health arena is one where money is everything. The apologists will say the welfare of those with bipolar is their main concern above everything else. The truth of the matter is those with bipolar are their main concern as long as they keep taking the drugs.

If one were to take the money out of the equation, it would be a different story. Bipolar disorder or manic depression or whatever you choose to call it is built on profit. Take that profit away and it would be a very different story. For example, research funding for some psychiatric drugs is being withdrawn as patents for particular drugs run out, and competing drug companies start to manufacture their own versions of the drug. The funding is being redirected into area where drug companies think the new blockbuster drug will come from. It goes without saying that in the psychiatric industry, money talks.

There is no question that people do experience problems and upsets in life that may result in mental troubles, sometimes very serious. But to say that these are 'mental illnesses' or caused by a 'chemical imbalance', like bipolar, that can only be treated with dangerous drugs is dishonest, harmful and often deadly. What psychiatric drugs do instead is mask the real cause of problems, often denying patients the opportunity to search for workable, effective, non-pharmaceutical solutions.

Many medical experts agree that an underlying physical illness could well explain emotional distress. The first step to take is to have a 'differential diagnosis', where the doctor obtains a thorough medical history and conducts a complete physical examination. In this way, he or she can rule out all problems that may cause a set of symptoms.

Remember, the mental health monopoly relies upon your ignorance of what is really going on. If you were fully informed, however, the potential of carrying on the psychiatric charade would be greatly diminished. It would also depend on what you chose to do with the information and whether you chose to act upon it, defend it or attack it. I began by saying people view life in different ways, from their own unique perspectives, with their own idiosyncratic thoughts on life, the universe and everything. After reading this preface, perhaps you will view current psychiatric practices from a different perspective, and perhaps you will recognise that a mental health monopoly is pulling the strings of our society and making us into psychiatric puppets. If you consider yourself to be more informed, and you wish to act, exert your power of choice and with your new-found wisdom, start cutting the strings.

Citations within Preface

1. http://www.ahrp.org/cms/content/view/828/9

2. http://voices.yahoo.com/equetro-fda-approved-treatment-bipolar-disorder-182290.html

3. http://www.nhs.uk/Conditions/Bipolar-disorder/Pages/Causes.aspx

4. http://www.pamf.org/teen/life/disorders/bipolar.html

5. http://www.cchrint.org/about-us/co-founder-dr-thomas-szasz/quotes-on-psychiatry-as-a-pseudo-science/

Part 1

The Bipolar Story

Introduction

We live in a world filled with beauty, wonderment and equilibrium – but equally one that is filled with evil, suffering and injustice. People with emotional and mental health problems have endured profound ignorance and bigotry from society for centuries.

'The Mad' have suffered for their difference more than most. Shunned and beaten as 'possessed by demons' in one age. Locked up and laughed at by crowds of tormenters in another. Subjected to barbarism beyond words in the name of quackery and science, and still today, in our bright and shiny, wonderful world, turned into living experiments, zombies and untouchables by poisons administered with smiles and gothic 'treatments' that leave them hardly sure of who they are.

They are 'The Mad.'

Except of course we do not call them mad any more. In the bright and shiny 20th and 21st centuries, we feel we must have explanations, diagnoses, labels. And so we slice up our society, and we give conditions names.

Bipolar is a name. A label. And that is all.

Bipolar is not a disease. You cannot catch it. More than that though – the list of symptoms that 'could indicate bipolar' is broad, and wide, and self-contradictory. As such, it is not a diagnosis of anything particular or concrete. It is potentially a catch-all of 'symptoms' that are not symptoms, and once 'diagnosed' it is like a snake that will slide you straight down to the dark side of our world, with little hope offered of escape or parole.

Of course, I do not mean to suggest that people do not get deeply, despairingly depressed, or that these same people, at different times, don't act in manic and dazzling and damaging ways. What I do claim is that these states are merely extreme manifestations of natural human responses to natural human difficulties associated with the business of being alive.

Look at our amazing world. In the last fifty years alone, medical science has advanced in awe-inspiring leaps and bounds. Incredible to think, then, that when it comes to bipolar, we're still treating supposed sufferers with poisonous and life-destroying drugs.

But my purpose here is not to start redefining bipolar. Rather, I want to help make people aware of the myths surrounding this alleged condition. I want to expose the unnecessary suffering inflicted through medication. And I want to develop a willingness in the reader to understand the facts about bipolar, and become more accustomed to looking at different methods of improving their emotional health, to which they have not given, or are not currently giving, enough attention.

Psychiatry has butchered its way through society for centuries in search of credibility, and instead of delivering the sanity it loftily promises, has bequeathed a legacy of utter wretchedness to those whose lives it has touched.

Of course, that's the point about 'The Mad'. That's why they've been more feared than any other group: they're the only group that's open to anyone, and the only group to which you can be consigned, against your will, on someone else's word. One misdiagnosis, one easy psychiatric solution, and you can find yourself on the chemical treadmill too.

That's why you need to read this book.

The Bipolar Story

Five important things you need to know about bipolar:

- There is no research in existence that conclusively proves that bipolar is a chemical imbalance in the brain.
- There is no research evidence that proves it a genetic condition.
- There are no research studies that accurately pinpoint its exact causes.
- There is no known cure; because doubts persist as to whether bipolar in its current psychiatric diagnostic context actually exists.
- Psychiatric and pharmaceutical companies work in partnership and make billions in profit by continuing to label people *bipolar* and unnecessarily medicating them.

International Classification of Diseases 10

In Britain, the manual used by psychiatrists to diagnose mental illnesses and disorders is called the *International Classification of Diseases* – commonly referred to as *ICD 10*, its present edition. In the case of bipolar, *ICD 10* lists signs and symptoms of mania. Patients must display symptoms deemed as manic for a period of at least one week. These include:

- Increased activity or physical restlessness.
- Flight of ideas or the subjective experience of thoughts racing.
- Loss of normal social inhibitions, resulting in behaviour that is inappropriate to the circumstances.
- Decreased need for sleep.
- Distractibility or constant changes in activity or plans.

According to *ICD 10*, depression must be present for a period of two weeks, along with the mania for one week, for a diagnosis of bipolar disorder to be made. Some of the symptoms listed in *ICD 10* for depression include:

- Lack of emotional reactions to events or activities that normally produce an emotional response.
- Waking in the morning two hours or more before the usual time.
- Depression worse in the morning.
- Marked loss of appetite and weight loss (5% or more of body weight in the past month).
- Marked loss of libido.

Millions of people around the world are fooled by the unproven and entirely hypothetical claim that bipolar is caused by a chemical imbalance in the brain. Without adequate scientific proof, bipolar cannot be accurately categorised as the disease of the brain that psychiatrists and the pharmaceutical companies claim it to be. After decades of trying to establish proof, they have failed to come up with anything remotely validating that claim – which therefore firmly remains a myth. Please reflect for a moment and consider that none of the following, for example, can prove what causes bipolar:

- brain scans
- blood tests
- DNA/genetic tests
- chemical imbalance tests
- X-rays
- any current laboratory tests not included above.

Please be 100% certain that there has been *no scientific research* or test carried out that has, even in the slightest – let alone unequivocally – proven that bipolar is carried by some kind of chemical imbalance or by any genetic family trait handed down from one generation to the next. As Soreff (2002) points out, 'There is no evidence of bipolar in the brain – no markers – no proof or evidence that it is genetic'. However, psychiatrists persist in stating that the problem lies in the brain and for whatever reason in their quest for a cure, be it gullibility or indifference, they continue to treat unsuspecting patients with mind-altering medication. While this is happening, the big pharmaceutical companies sit back and make billions.

Psychiatric diagnoses are completely subjective and have no scientific or medical validity. Whereas real diseases, like cancer or diabetes, are discovered in labs, psychiatric disorders are invented by being voted into existence by medical committee members from their scant subjective view of symptoms, which they judge to be sufficient to label someone with a mental illness, like bipolar.

The lists of characteristics used to describe mania and depression in this psychiatric bible are neither clever nor profound and most people who have never even heard of bipolar will be able to identify moments of their lives when they've had instances of mania or depression. And that's about all that *ICD 10* consists of: lists of feelings and behavioural traits, because in the absence of valid scientific research – and the inability to carry out blood and other biological tests that can ascertain the presence or absence of a mental illness – the only source available to psychiatrists is empirical data and at best this remains a subjective guessing game.

What causes bipolar disorder?

The cause is unknown, but it is clear that those with the condition experience a plethora of difficult life situations. Bipolar is most probably caused or closely linked to a traumatic life event. This could be a singular trauma or a series of traumatic events, the culmination of which is extreme emotional stress and psychological overload. Traumatic events might include childhood abuse, the death of a loved one, relationship difficulties, bullying, financial problems, or indeed any other stressful change in life patterns. These factors are sometimes fuelled by alcohol and drug misuse mistakenly intended to alleviate the stress, but ultimately the end result is a further disintegration of life, ranging from relationship breakdowns and family disruption to unemployment, bankruptcy, social isolation and suicidal behaviour. It is clear that those affected by the condition have not had the resources needed to adequately deal with the challenging situations that have led to these difficulties.

Somewhere in the person's life will lay the root cause which ultimately alters their moods and perspective on life. Such chronically stressful situations can cause a person to develop an erratic personality. This, coupled with taking illegal drugs, alcohol abuse and psychiatric medication, interferes with the emotional functioning of the person. Difficulties usually start in early adulthood but there are sometimes problems in adolescence that can cause irrational moods to develop earlier, for example, young people with behavioural difficulties, those with poor academic functioning or those who experience abuse, post-traumatic stress disorder or family difficulties, along with substance/alcohol misuse.

Others signs and symptoms of bipolar

We are led to believe that the construction of bipolar has two completely opposite sets of symptoms. It is a serious behavioural and mood disorder with debilitating consequences in which a person experiences bouts of mania lasting days, weeks or months – alternating with long periods of depression. It consists of periods of mania where the person experiences increased physical activity, high levels of energy, distractibility and irritability. For months, even years, the person's mood is otherwise perfectly normal. The term bipolar refers to people experiencing both extremes of mood.

Although everybody has mood swings to some degree, the depth and intensity of moods in the bipolar person are extreme and prolonged. These mood swings disturb the everyday patterns of living to an immense degree.

Just imagine someone who at the beginning of the week is dashing around with super strength and speed. This person will want to take on the biggest job and will have great plans for completing the most impossible task. They will become irritable and aggressive with those who don't share in their interest. They will be unable to sleep, so great are their energy levels – resulting in thoughts of being invincible, coupled with paranoia and hallucinations affecting their vision or perception.

Other signs and symptoms of the manic phase are:

- Delusions or hallucinations relating to grandiose ideas about religion, politics and creativity.
- Non-stop talkativeness with domineering and provocative behaviour.
- High sexual desire verging on promiscuity.
- Spending foolishly – sometimes running up massive debt.

Manic episodes consist of high bursts of energy and creativity – often delusional and combined with reckless behaviours including promiscuity and over-spending. These chaotic activities, coupled with sleep deprivation and lack of food and water, create a toxic state in the human body, resulting in a metabolic burn-out.

On the opposite end of the scale to manic episodes are recurring cycles of depression. People living with bipolar will experience deep depression, where they stay in bed for days or weeks. They experience a total lack of interest in life, lack of energy and motivation to do even the simplest of things, like taking a shower or brushing their teeth. This will be coupled with feelings of worthlessness and hopelessness (as opposed to sadness). This will be followed by a deep and foreboding sense of pessimism, which sometimes leads to suicidal thoughts.

Other signs and symptoms of the depressed phase are:

- A persistent anxious feeling coupled with feeling pessimistic about everything.
- Total loss of interest in work and leisure activities – and sex.
- Reduced or increased appetite.
- Poor concentration and indecision along with being delusional, having hallucinations and disturbed or illogical thinking.

We all have our ups and downs, our 'on' and 'off' days, but with bipolar disorder these peaks and valleys are more severe. The symptoms of the condition ruin academic and employment performance, damage relationships and disrupt daily life. But there are ways to stop this from happening, which I shall come onto later in this book. You will discover ways of curtailing, stabilising and managing this condition. But firstly, it is important to learn what the symptoms look like, because recognising the problem is the first step to getting it under control. The people featured in the *Life Stories* in this book all recount traumatic experiences which changed their personalities and moods. One of the contributors summed up bipolar rather succinctly:

When I'm in a manic phase, I feel as though I am capable of anything and everything. This can be an amazing feeling, but I sometimes get frustrated and angry with people. Ideas flow constantly and quickly, as if my brain is on fast-forward. Everything happening in the world has significance in my life. But when I'm depressed, it's as if I'm completely crushed and living in slow motion. I feel capable of nothing.

Psychiatrists routinely do not inform patients of non-drug treatments, nor do they conduct thorough *medical* examinations to ensure that a person's problem does not stem from an untreated medical condition manifesting as 'psychiatric' symptoms. They do not accurately inform patients of the nature of the diagnoses, which would require informing the patient that psychiatric diagnoses are completely subjective and based on a list of behaviours. Furthermore, contemporary psychiatric practice is about reducing manic and depressive symptoms instead of looking at the emotional state or cultural diversity of the person. Psychiatrists therefore classify bipolar according to the symptoms and medicate their patients to conform to what they consider to be normal behaviour, without considering their individuality, ethnic background, gender, race and other diverse factors.

It is well known by professionals working in the arena of mental health that misdiagnosis is rampant because sustained periods of the presenting symptoms have not been determined. The other obvious reason is there is no test, no scan and no scientific measure for a mood disorder – therefore a poorly trained psychiatrist is highly likely to misdiagnose. I can never understand why people do not seek a second or third opinion instead of settling for an imprisoning diagnosis at the first hurdle – which often then automatically subjects them to a lifetime of medication.

Categories of bipolar

Bipolar I disorder

This is the classic form of the illness when the person has recurrent episodes of mania and depression but is mainly characterised by the manic episodes. Generally this manic period is followed by a period of depression, although some bipolar I individuals may not experience a major depressive episode. All of the *Life Stories* or people referred to in this book will fall into this category.

Bipolar II disorder

This is when there are longer lasting major depressive episodes alternating with episodes of hypomania, which is characterised by an elevated or irritable mood with bursts of energy but is a much milder form of the condition than bipolar I, because people with bipolar II will never have experienced a full-blown manic episode. It may not affect an individual's ability to function on a day-to-day basis.

Rapid cycling bipolar disorder

This diagnosis may be given when an individual's mood fluctuates rapidly and is characterised by four or more mood episodes that occur within a 12-month period. Some people experience multiple episodes within a single week, or even within a single day. A rapid cycling pattern increases the risk of severe depression and suicidal tendencies.

Mixed bipolar disorder state

This is when people have symptoms of mania and depression at the same time in what is called a mixed bipolar state. These often include agitation, trouble sleeping and change in appetite, psychosis and suicidal thinking. A person may have a very sad, hopeless mood while at the same time feeling extremely energised.

Bipolar statistics

Statistics for bipolar are as unreliable as the diagnostic criteria for the condition. It is unlikely you will ever read the same facts and figures twice that corroborate a realistic picture of the 'condition'. Here is a selection I have collected from a wide spectrum of books, journals, newspapers and websites.

Until a few decades ago, bipolar was considered a rare illness; the *World Health Organization* now considers it as one of the top causes of lost years of life and health in 15–44 year olds, ranking above war, violence and schizophrenia. Other statistics suggest:

- Between 10 and 20% of people with bipolar have rapid cycling, although women comprise 70–90% of this.

- 30% of people diagnosed with bipolar will have serious drug and alcohol misuse issues in their lives. Illicit drugs, like cannabis, cocaine, ecstasy and amphetamines, can cause either depression or mania in people who are predisposed to mood-swings.
- Bipolar disorder is recurrent, meaning that more than 90% of individuals who have a single manic episode will go on to experience future episodes.
- Roughly 70% of manic episodes in bipolar disorder occur immediately before or after a depressive episode.
- People from lower socio-economic backgrounds are eight times more likely to be given a diagnosis of bipolar.
- Bipolar is between ten and forty times more common among artists than among the general public.
- People who take antidepressants are three times more likely to attempt suicide or succeed in killing themselves.

The UK-based *Equilibrium Bipolar Foundation* states that bipolar probably affects up to one out of every hundred adults in the world. Other statistics suggest:

- 2.4 million people in the UK have bipolar.
- Twice as many women as men get diagnosed with the condition.
- Women are more prone to depressive episodes – while men, who by nature are generally less passive than women, will have more manic episodes,

although the gender ratio of those with the condition is equal.

- Some people receive a range of diagnoses before bipolar is determined, with this often taking up to ten years.
- Bipolar increases the risk of suicide by up to twenty times. Between 25 and 50% of people with bipolar attempt suicide at least once.
- Even with current medical treatments, people with bipolar spend around 50% of their lives after onset with significant symptoms, mainly depressive.
- Fewer than 10% of people are ever offered Cognitive Behavioural Therapy or any other talking therapy as part of their recovery plan.

Aware Ireland suggests that bipolar affects men and women equally – that it can affect anyone from presidents to porters – and that 40,000 people in Ireland live with the condition. However, the Department of Psychiatry at the *National University of Ireland, Galway*, claims that bipolar affects 100,000 people in Ireland. According to research carried out by the *Boyne Research Institute,* the average age of diagnosis in Ireland is 34.5 years – and for many people with the condition a major life event had coincided with the onset of symptoms, such as giving birth or the break-up of a relationship. Other statistics suggest:

- 15% of relatives of bipolar patients have a serious mood disorder.
- The causes of bipolar are 70% genetic and 30% due to environmental factors.

- 75% of patients are effectively treated with Lithium, although only 30% of those with rapid cycling bipolar are successfully treated with the same agent.
- 80% of patients will experience a relapse of bipolar if they suddenly withdraw from Lithium.
- Only 5% of people with bipolar have manic episodes that are not followed by depression, however, if a person has only one episode of depression or mania, there is a 50% chance that neither will occur.
- 75% of people with bipolar smoke cigarettes compared to 23% of the general population.

Charting the history of bipolar

Little changes in the world of mental health. Unlike conventional medicine, there have been no major medical breakthroughs that have produced a scientific answer to what causes bipolar or what cures it. Progress is still so minimal that its methods of diagnosis and treatment have remained those of amateurs for well over a hundred years – methods that are at best negligible and at worst cause premature death, owing to the catalogue of damage done to the body's central nervous system and organs by the unrelenting regime of harsh medication. But where did this terrible fallacy first begin? Let's take a look at a snapshot picture of its origins and see how bipolar has evolved within this mindset in the last fifty years.

As you have already read, bipolar is not a disease or some germ that can be seen at first under a microscope. This false label, which psychiatrists have given the condition, has no scientific basis and is not a medical condition because if it were, it would come under the realm of traditional medicine and not under psychiatry. But you have to go back and look at the origins of psychiatry to understand why we have arrived at the point at which we now find ourselves. The birthplace of psychiatry is Germany where it started in the late 1800s. Professor Wundt, a psychologist and philosopher was one of the first of his contemporaries to become fascinated with the psyche – the human soul – and decided to carry out research in this field. He wanted to know how the soul worked, and tried to quantify and show how it was put together. When he couldn't find any answers as to what the soul actually was, he covered this up and simply proclaimed that the soul didn't exist.

Freud, the Austrian neurologist who founded psycho-analysis around the same time as Wundt was busy in his clinic, fared little better. He believed that all humans were born perverse, with dark hidden thoughts in their minds from the very beginning, claiming that dialogue with a trained person was the only way to release these demons buried deep within the unconscious. But Freud was a great advocate of cocaine and publicly recommended the drug, which resulted in most of his discoveries being tarnished as those of a cocaine psychosis, as he self-medicated with the drug to treat his depression. Freud was obsessed with libido, sex and incest – with his greatest fascination being sexual abuse, claiming his most disturbed patients were those who held unconscious memories of sexual abuse in infancy. However, as Webster (1995) stated, Freud later confirmed he had no proof to back up this claim, admitting that he may have misinterpreted fantasies as actual facts from his patients.

Asylums were created between the seventeenth and nineteenth centuries to treat people who were considered mentally ill. People who experienced hallucinations, were deemed peculiar, had learning disabilities or were anxious, manic and depressed, were all incarcerated with each other – often for the remainder of their lives. There were only two official diagnoses back then – schizophrenia and depression. A form of Valium was the only medication usually used to treat both conditions. What is remarkable about this is that currently we have over 400 mental disorders in the *ICD 10* diagnostic manual and still psychiatrists treat all of these conditions, including bipolar, with the same antipsychotic medication used to treat a variety of other conditions. Indeed little has changed, leaving the route of progress open for pioneering research and results, both of which are slow in coming forth.

1930s & 1940s

Doctors claimed that manic patients would calm down after a while by themselves with little interference from the medical profession. This conservative approach came with the advice for patients to get plenty of fresh air, hot baths and bed rest. Sedative drugs were used in extreme and prolonged cases of mania. But this sensible approach wasn't pleasing to all psychiatrists and further meddling led to the use of Electroconvulsive therapy (ECT). Psychiatrists thought that the best case results of using ECT were found in patients with both mania and depression. ECT was first introduced in 1938 by Italian neuropsychiatrists Ugo Cerletti and Lucio Bini, and gained widespread use as a form of treatment between the 1940s and 1960s for a variety of conditions, including epilepsy. It consists of passing an electrical current through the brain to produce an epileptic fit – hence the name, electroconvulsive.

These electrically induced seizures in anesthetised patients were first tested on pigs, before Cerletti started using the technique on his patients, alleging that these electric shocks caused his obsessive and difficult mental patients to become meek and manageable. However, it was soon noticed that there were no long-term benefits of ECT because patients felt no better a few weeks after having it than before. Instead, many felt more disorientated as a result, coupled with impaired attention, memory loss, epileptic fits and in some cases, lasting brain damage. Before antipsychotics and Lithium were known about, ECT was used to treat mania. It is still used to the present day on patients with prolonged depression who are suicidal. As well as causing memory loss and persistent apathy, ECT results in seizures – which is ironic because it was created in the belief that it in fact *prevented* seizures. Victims of ECT never recover their original selves because healthy cells in the brain are mutilated during the course of this barbaric procedure.

1950s

Every time the word *Lithium* (Camcolit, Liskonum, Priadel, and Li-liquid) appears in the media, it is automatically recognised as a drug that is taken for bipolar, particularly for the treatment of mania. John Cade, an Australian psychiatrist, discovered it in the fifties. Lithium is a ground metal extracted from natural sources and combined as a salt as either a carbonate or citrate and made into a substance that can be taken as a medicine. Given the sedation associated with its neurological toxicity, Lithium can be predicted to reduce levels of excitement and activity in people with acute mania. It is profoundly toxic to the human body in relatively small doses. While Lithium is still routinely prescribed as a mood stabiliser, it is not known how the substance works to combat mania. Although non-addictive, it is dangerous to withdraw from Lithium, as the nervous system will react with an episode of mania/psychosis. However, if it is given or taken in high doses (which often occurs) it has the same harsh side-effects as those received from taking antipsychotic medication and antidepressants. Psychiatrists insist that it can take up to two years to reach its full effect as a mood stabiliser and that if it doesn't completely stop mood swings, it usually reduces their severity. But many people with bipolar are kept on it for life to prevent mania recurring. The problem with Lithium is that a certain level of the drug has to be produced in the blood for it to be effective. But if the level rises too much, unpleasant and potentially serious side-effects can occur including:

- tremors
- unsteadiness
- weight gain
- diarrhoea
- slurred speech
- drowsiness

- blurred vision
- urinating more frequently
- swollen ankles
- a slow-down in thinking
- headaches
- muscle aches
- problems with the thyroid gland
- fits and unconsciousness.

But, ultimately, problems with the thyroid gland may cause psychotic symptoms that resemble mania or depression. The toxicity of Lithium is very dangerous. Lithium salts have a narrow therapeutic and toxic ratio and require regular blood tests to measure Lithium levels and also to monitor for heart, thyroid and kidney abnormalities.

Taking Lithium in pregnancy has shown abnormalities in babies and can cause cardiac birth defects. It also gets into breast milk, making it highly dangerous for newborn babies. Lithium also has potentially serious interactions with a number of prescribed drugs (for example, steroids for asthma and medication for high blood pressure).

Two out of every three people with bipolar will be on Lithium at some point in their lives but these days it is rarely used as the only treatment for acute mania, which illustrates a practical acknowledgement of its limitations, and is invariably taken as an adjunct to antipsychotics and/or antidepressants. In addition to the side-effects already listed, Lithium taken with antipsychotic drugs leads to muscular disorders and has poisonous effects on the central nervous system. When taken with antidepressants, it attacks the central nervous system and leads to convulsions.

On the subject of the latter, antipsychotics were first discovered in the 1950s (more about these later). Also introduced around the same time were antidepressants which later became known as 'tricyclics'. These were in circulation for forty years until they were replaced by newer brands which were supposedly more sophisticated and more effective at producing serotonin levels in the brain. Side-effects of tricyclics included hair loss, bladder problems and constant drowsiness (placing patients in a *zombie* like state). They also carried a greater risk of cardiovascular disease such as heart attack or stroke. Although tricyclics are less frequently used in current times, they are still occasionally prescribed in the UK with the most popular types being the following:

1. Imipramine (Tofranil)
2. Dosulepin (Prothiaden, Dothep, Thaden and Dopress)
3. Amitriptyline (Tryptomer, Elavil, Tryptizol, Laroxyl)
4. Nortriptyline (Sensoval, Aventyle, Pamelor, Norpress)
5. Doxepin (Sinequan).

1960s & 1970s

Sedatives began to be freely prescribed in this era, more than at any point ever before in medical history. Little by little these drugs over the years have become common place, getting prescribed to ease the throes of manic episodes or to suppress tendencies of mania before they allegedly set into patients 'predisposed' to such symptoms. In current times, they are given in the form of Benzodiazepines, such as: Diazepam (Valium, Diastat) and Lorazepam (Ativan).

The side effects of these may include:

- drowsiness, unusual tiredness or weakness or feeling like you might pass out
- muscle spasm or muscle weakness
- blurred or double vision
- constipation or diarrhoea
- dryness of mouth or increased thirst
- increased bronchial secretions or watering of mouth
- nausea or vomiting
- problems with urination or loss of bladder control
- trembling or shaking
- drooling or dry mouth or slurred speech
- confusion, hallucinations, unusual thoughts or behaviour
- unusual risk-taking behaviour, decreased inhibitions or no fear of danger
- depressed mood, thoughts of suicide or hurting yourself.

In addition to sedatives the usage of antipsychotics had gathered momentum and allowed physiatrists to claim that they could successfully treat patients in their own communities, as opposed to keeping them locked up in asylums.

Haloperidol and Chlorpromazine were the two main antipsychotic drugs used in this approach. The government at the time supported this 'medical' model approach and so the process of closing asylums began. Psychiatrists went mainstream, spreading the myth that bipolar was caused by a chemical imbalance in the brain in an attempt to gain a respectable status for their profession. But the public weren't informed by the psychiatric profession of the now notorious side-effects that came with these new medications, which those with the condition gladly took in the hope of a cure. The list of side-effects is mesmerising, especially as all antipsychotic medication is toxic to both the heart and the central nervous system. It invariably leads to substantial weight gain, diabetes, brain atrophy, neurological impairment and increases the risk of coronary heart disease and cardiovascular disorder such as a stroke.

Here is a list of the adverse side-effects from each of these drugs.

Haloperidol (Haldol, Dozic, Serenace):

- weight gain
- muscle stiffness and cramping
- tremors
- involuntary mouth movements
- restlessness
- metabolic disruption
- depression, severe enough to result in suicide.

Chlorpromazine (Largactil):

- weight gain
- agitation
- tiredness

- breathing difficulties
- muscle spasms
- severe and persistent constipation
- bruising and bleeding
- liver problems.

Psychiatrists back in the sixties and seventies told their patients that an unfortunate aspect to taking medication that controls bipolar was the side-effects – or implied that the side-effects were in actual fact attributable to bipolar itself.

The myth of antipsychotics consisted of psychiatrists saying that these drugs incorporated the idea of there being a specific treatment to offer for bipolar. There were even those who claimed bipolar could be approached in essentially the same way as physical illness, but in the absence of the medical structure and the research findings to declare this as factual, the fallacy remained intact.

1980s

Although the term bipolar was first used in the fifties to differentiate unipolar depression from bipolar depression, the name change did not take place until 1980. The third edition of the *Diagnostic and Statistical Manual of Mental Disorders (DSM)* determined that the term *manic depression* be officially changed and replaced in the classification system to *bipolar disorder*.

However, the term *manic depression* is still widely used today by many to describe the condition. For some people it clearly states what the condition actually *is* in straightforward words, i.e. the term is plain and simple and its definition is self-explanatory. But others feel the term is stigmatising, with popular phrases such as 'Manic Monday' having crept into everyday colloquial language and in lyrics to songs.

But in the last few decades the psychiatric profession has made a concerted effort to shift the name change into mainstream language. They believe bipolar disorder is more of a clinical term, less emotionally loaded. It was also felt *manic depression* was incorrectly used to describe depression in general – including clinical depression. It was believed bipolar allowed for more clarity in a diagnosis because of its emphasis on the predominant symptoms of both manic and depressive characteristics.

1990s & 2000s

Bipolar was originally only an adult diagnosis but during the 1990s it started to appear in America as a child diagnosis as well. Since then it has gathered momentum, just like ADHD has over the years. In fact, the new edition of DSM 5 has devoted an entire section to the diagnosis. This is very worrying because, although this is not a diagnosis currently given to children in the UK and Ireland or indeed anywhere else in Europe, it needs to be monitored. It is easy to see how we might arrive at a point in the future where its use has become common practice and then one day, as in the story of ADHD, people could turn around and question, 'How come there was none of this twenty years ago?'

Mood stabilisers came into the frame in the middle 1990s and remain to be seen as profitable by pharmaceutical companies. Those widely used include:

1.   Sodium Valproate/Semisodium (Depakote)
2.   Lamotrigine (Lamictal)
3.   Carbamazepine (Tegretol).

All of these have a range of debilitating side-effects including:

• aching joints or muscles
• constipation and/or diarrhoea
• dryness of mouth and irritation or soreness of tongue
  or mouth
• headaches
• skin problems
• increased sweating
• loss of appetite
• loss of hair
• erectile dysfunction and lowering of sperm count
• stomach pain or discomfort.

New antipsychotic drugs were introduced in the 1990s under the collective heading 'atypical' as opposed to the earlier ones in the 1950s which were labelled 'typical'. A combination of the older drugs and newer ones are still widely prescribed today. After the introduction of the newer antipsychotics, in some cases people with mild signs of mania or depression were encouraged to start taking this medication, supposedly as a deterrent to prevent symptoms of bipolar emerging later in life. The most widely used of these 'atypical' drugs are:

1.   Olanzapine (Zyprexa)
2.   Risperidone (Risperdal)
3.   Quetiapine (Seroquel XL)
4.   Aripiprazole (Abilify).

These second generation drugs are marketed as having apparently less serious side-effects that the older types, but readers will fail to understand how the harrowing side-effects of the 'new' medications can be described as less debilitating than, for example, Haloperidol and Chlorpromazine were in previous decades.

The side-effects of these 'new' drugs are mesmerising and include:

- impaired judgement, thinking and motor skills
- increased appetite and weight gain
- irritability
- aggression and violence
- sedation
- constipation and haemorrhoids (piles) and/or diarrhoea
- urinary retention
- apathy, lack of emotion
- erectile disfunction, delayed ejaculation and lack of orgasm (men)
- failure to achieve orgasm/delayed orgasm (women)
- low or high blood pressure
- muscle pain and tremors
- hypersalivation
- photosensitivity
- constant drowsiness
- abdominal pain
- dizzy spells
- sluggishness
- inflammation or swelling of the sinuses

- suicidal ideation
- sudden death.

As established in research carried out by Petry (2008), Raphael (2009) and in a large study carried out by the National Association of State Mental Health Programme Directors in Canada (2006), it is not uncommon for people to die in their early forties because of these serious health conditions. Putting a foreign substance, such as an antipsychotic, into the body disrupts the body's normal biochemistry. Sometimes this disruption creates a false and temporary feeling of euphoria. The result does not last. The drugs just mask the problem. Patients end up having their dosages increased to maintain this false sense of well-being. Higher dosages or changes to other medications ultimately lead to addiction.

These new antipsychotics were marketed as having fewer side-effects than the first generation antipsychotics but this is in the main another falsehood, because they still contribute to metabolic side-effects such as weight gain/obesity, cardiovascular disease, diabetes and respiratory problems, increased glucose and lipids as well as weakened immunity. They also fail to bring about change in reduced motivation and emotional expressiveness. Because each medication (whether first or second generation) has its own profile of desirable and adverse effects, a psychiatrist may recommend one of the older *typical* or newer *atypical* antipsychotics alone or in combination with other medications (e.g. Lithium and antidepressants).

Antidepressants

Antidepressants, too, as a disease-specific treatment are not validated by any scientific evidence that proves that bipolar is caused by malfunctioning neurotransmitters or chemical imbalances in the brain. However, psychiatrists from the late 1950s to the present day have falsely led people to believe that the depressive aspect of bipolar can only be treated through medication; hence they freely prescribe antidepressants. But instead of people showing signs of recovery, adverse effects appear with the following characteristics:

- Dulled senses and blunted emotions.
- Greater feelings of hopelessness and powerlessness than before taking the medication, which considerably increases the risk of suicide.
- Moods may become more unstable than prior to taking them.
- They also prevent people from working through their problems or building inner resilience which helps them face future problems with greater strength and determination.

The newer types of antidepressants were introduced in the early 1990s, and were known as Selective Serotonin Reuptake Inhibitors (SSRIs). These more expensive drugs mainly replaced traditional tricyclics which had been around since the fifties and supposedly improved tolerability.

The older tricyclics were believed to work on two neurotransmitters in the brain – serotonin and norepinephrine – but were also believed to cause patients being treated with depression to switch from this to mania in over 25% of cases.

SSRIs are selective because they act only on one neurotransmitter in the brain – serotonin. It is believed that normal levels of serotonin are required to regulate moods and other functions. Slowing the release of serotonin from the brain is thought to improve moods and other functions. But a big disadvantage of SSRIs for many was that they were alleged to be less effective in treating depression and bipolar than the older tricyclics.

The most common SSRI antidepressants in use today are:

1. Citalopram (Celexa)
2. Fluoxetine (Prozac)
3. Paroxetine (Seroxat)
4. Escitopram (Lexapro)
5. Sertraline (Zoloft).

Despite the clever marketing by pharmaceutical companies promoting fewer side-effects to these drugs, the reality proved otherwise, with the more notable ones being:

- insomnia
- ejaculation problems
- nausea
- weakness
- headache
- diarrhoea
- loss of appetite
- drowsiness
- anxiety
- nervousness
- shakiness (tremors)

- dry mouth
- decreased sex drive
- yawning
- indigestion
- dizziness
- sweating
- impotence
- fatigue
- slow heartbeat
- rapid heartbeat
- neck/jaw pain
- flu-like symptoms
- all over body pain
- hot flashes
- pins and needles feeling in head/extremities
- weight gain
- abdominal pain
- tiredness/lack of energy
- numbness
- emotional numbness
- irritability
- akathisia (uncontrollable limb and body movements, severe restlessness)
- suicide.

Antidepressants are mood altering elevators, with some brands becoming known during the nineties as 'liquid sunshine' because of their uplifting and sometimes euphoric effect. However, street drugs like cocaine and amphetamines also have a similar effect, yet society in the main clearly admonishes illicit drug use and would never for a second condone people taking illegal substances to alleviate mental distress. They would know this is not the correct way to go about solving the underlying emotional problem. Yet society wears blinkers when it comes to antidepressants and other psychiatric drugs – although they cause the same lasting damage as illegal street drugs.

Suicidal feelings

Taking antidepressants may make some people feel suicidal when they had not considered this before they started the medication. Suicidal feelings have mainly been associated with SSRIs. It has been noted that the ability to summon up motivation for suicide is intensified after an initial course of SSRI antidepressants because of a shift in thinking, which makes the person more likely to act on their compulsion to end their life.

Serotonin Syndrome

This is serious and potentially fatal *effect* of antidepressants. It may occur with any antidepressant, but is more likely with SSRIs, especially if they are given with other psychiatric drugs and Lithium. It may come on very suddenly. Its symptoms are, (most common first):

- headache
- feeling sick
- diarrhoea
- high temperature, shivering, sweating
- high blood pressure, fast heart rate

- tremor, muscle twitching, over-responsive reflexes
- convulsions (fits)
- agitation, confusion, hallucinations
- loss of consciousness (coma)
- addiction to antidepressants.

Some people become 'tolerant' to antidepressants after taking them for some time and have to increase the dosage to maintain the original effect. Addiction is commonplace, in addition to withdrawal symptoms if abruptly stopped, resulting in many having to go back on them. If you have been taking antidepressants for a long time, you may also develop a psychological dependency on them. Taking antidepressants in pregnancy increases the risk of miscarriage and of congenital problems as well as premature birth. There is evidence that taking SSRIs early in pregnancy slightly increases the risk of heart defects, spina bifida, cleft palate and hare lip as outlined in a revised booklet issued by the mental health charity *Mind* (Darton 2011). New forms of antidepressants have been seen to cause people to display symptoms of emotional apathy and indifference never seen before in humankind and, for some, this will also have meant a steep increase in both the risk of suicidal thinking, and of suicide itself.

Damage caused by medication

As previously mentioned, antidepressants and other psychiatric medication attack both the central nervous system and immune system. The body is a magnificent piece of machinery – made up of over a hundred trillion cells that are all linked together. Every cell in the body will be affected by antidepressants and antipsychotic medications. The immune system is a very intelligent and proactive mechanism that will react to the damage caused by the medication because it will recognise that what is occurring in the body is caused by an outside agent, as the receptor sights for these medications are situated outside the central nervous system. People have various levels of serotonin in their bodies but when they take antidepressants the body can shut down its natural ability to create its own. Should we be disrupting nature this way when the long-term consequences are not yet known?

Research and publications

Vietal and Phillips (2007) examined the validity of bipolar as a diagnostic category owing to the ambiguity of its diagnosis but critiques like this often get quickly suppressed by psychiatrics and rarely gain publicity or prominance.

Although governments in the UK and Ireland have acknowledged that the economic burden of mental illness cannot be tackled without proper research investment, little ever gets done beyond the rhetoric. It angers me that I do not have any significant research findings to report here that would cast better understanding on what causes bipolar.

Instead, there are hundreds of mediocre papers available and if you want to delve into the field of psychiatric research a little more, one of the best books available that gives an insightful and balanced critique about psychiatric research is, in my opinion, *The Myth of the Chemical Cure* by Dr Joanna Moncrieff. Here you will see the findings of small scale studies of which many exist noting minor improvements between patients who take psychiatric medication and those taking a placebo.

I personally will only get excited when psychiatric research is conducted and it concludes with a possible cause or cure of bipolar – or both – that does not involve psychotropic drugs. Indeed, how great it would be if there was research available which showed that psychiatric medication does not attack the central nervous system, or have debilitating side-effects, is not addictive or destructive and ultimately does not lead to an early death.

Now that's wishful thinking.

Although universities generally encourage free speech, one needs to question whether the teachings and findings of faculties of pharmacology, medicine and mental health, which are heavily funded by large pharmaceutical companies, are impartial and do not have connotations of invested interest. This would also be true of medical journals. I have spoken to professionals who either had great difficulty or were outright refused to have their studies peer reviewed or published in medical journals. The simple truth is that pharmaceutical companies are loath to fund or provide research that will be used to educate or advertise alternatives to psychotropic drugs. Could it be that anything or anyone who poses a threat of putting the slightest dent in pharmaceutical profits will be shunned?

I have also found during my research that it is easy to formulate the thought that psychiatrists will go out on a limb to point out that they are disadvantaged because of not having medical tests to rely upon, which other doctors readily have at their disposal when diagnosing physical diseases. Take any book on bipolar that is prefixed with the title *Living with*, *Coping with* or *Life with* – you too are more than likely to discover that the author is a psychiatrist that will demonstrate profound arrogance to convince you that, in the absence of these tests, their expertise has to be greater than that of medical doctors because of having to rely on sound judgement to diagnose the different mental illnesses outlined in the diagnostic manuals.

The dwindling spiral

Bipolar is saturated with myths, with some people believing only artists, writers and musicians get bipolar. In fact, millions of people from all walks of life experience these abnormal shifts in mood, from deep depression to elation, from thoughts of grandeur to thoughts of hopelessness, from an abundance of energy to lethargy. You will see later in the *Life Stories* from the people who I interviewed for this book, how they refer to their fluctuating moods that often makes it impossible for them to function properly – often resulting in an inability to work, coupled with poor life skills, risky behaviours, relationship difficulties and drug and alcohol problems. When these manifestations are presented before a psychiatrist, they will consult their checklists, diagnose bipolar and then start their patient on a lifelong journey of medication. There is little time for patients to be listened to, invested in or understood – nor is there any other alternative explored, apart from antidepressants, antipsychotics, Lithium, mood stabilisers and sleeping tablets. Psychiatric medication compounds the initial problem to phenomenal heights because of its debilitating side-effects, which turn into chronic and life-threatening illnesses of their own accord, and can result in the worst effect – death itself, by suicide.

One might say when a person sees a psychiatrist and starts taking medication, this becomes the moment he or she enters the pathway of the dwindling spiral that is often coupled with the revolving door syndrome where patients are continuously in and out of hospital. They become embroiled in a system that promises them they'll get better but fails to deliver, until one day they arrive at a point where they have become detached from the world, and where the world no longer recognises them as an individual. How can you call any society that allows this to happen to its people responsible?

Very few psychiatrists really understand how the drugs work or the side-effects they are going to have on anyone. It still depends on the luck of the draw which drug is going to be tolerable. Take two people – Billy and Jack. One drug works for Billy, but completely obliterates Jack's social skills. Do you blame the psychiatrist or is it a reality that we have to accept? There are no magic pills that treat bipolar. There is no one prescription that fits all. It is merely an academic exercise. With antipsychotic medication you solve one problem – e.g. a manic episode, for a short period of time – but the next thing you know you end up with two problems. The treatment turns a period of crisis into a chronic and enduring health problem. Regrettably, psychiatrists don't appear to recognise that it is the body's reaction to the drugs and not the drugs' action on the body that causes unwanted side-effects. That is why the drugs affect each and every one of us differently. If your body is more sensitive than mine, or less tolerant, it is likely you will have more debilitating side-effects than I will endure. But psychiatrists fail to acknowledge this varyingly toxic effect and will meddle with the dosages or mix different medications together in the hope of greater tolerance. Instead this invariably only intensifies the situation. This could explain why some people can take a drug for some weeks, months or years and not be too badly affected while others can become debilitatingly sick, irritable, hostile, suicidal and even homicidal (although every person's central nervous system will endure damage irrespective of the level of side-effects that individually appear). It's our unique bodies' reaction to the drugs and not the other way around. In that sense, taking drugs for bipolar is like playing Russian roulette: you don't know when or what reaction you're going to get, but rest assured, it is only a matter of time. Ultimately, few can tell when 'bipolar' ends and medication takes over, thus making it difficult to know what are real emotional manifestations and what symptoms are medication induced?

Conclusion

Getting a diagnosis of bipolar is something to avoid because there is nothing good about having this disorder. It becomes for many an endless cycle of taking medications that cause bad side-effects as well as deteriorating health, sometimes leading to an early death. A better understanding of the variance of moods is necessary to avoid the pitfalls caused by not understanding periods of high activity or depressive moments – and learning to modify moods through adequate diet, exercise and sleep. There are some people though who suspect they are bipolar – or who have been given a diagnosis but refuse to take medication, opting instead to monitor their moods by avoiding stressful situations and by living a healthy lifestyle that is devoid of alcohol and illicit drugs.

Part 2

Life Stories

Introduction

Imagine you knew nothing about the flu. Imagine the flu was still exotic, poorly understood and shrouded in some medical mystery. When you went to your doctor, you'd be scared, you'd be worried, and you'd probably take your doctor's word for it when they told you of a cure or a treatment, whatever it entailed. The feeling of illness and the shroud of mystery would make you put your life and your health entirely in their hands.

Welcome to the world of bipolar.

As we have seen, the 'symptoms' of bipolar are many, varied and self-contradictory. Any two-bit snake-oil salesman could come along with a miracle cure, and people with a diagnosis of bipolar would have little option (and often no option at all) but to take it. But of course, two-bit snake-oil salesmen wouldn't be allowed to operate by governments, and they wouldn't have access to sufferers in need.

Pharmaceutical companies in the 21st century are no two-bit snake-oil salesmen. They preside over a truly colossal industry, which dictates the health of millions and the careers of research scientists across the globe. They subsidise hospitals in exchange for promotion of their latest miracle, they sponsor research to prove those miracles work, and they have, through a highly-paid and terrifyingly effective lobbying network and through job creation potential, the ability to influence health policy on a massive scale. These are untouchable snake-oil salesmen in very, very fine suits, who also – through funding and connections in the psychiatric profession, have almost mandatory access to a customer base for their products. Psychiatry essentially puts patients on a conveyor belt and delivers them, hands out and mouths open, to the machinations of Big Pharma.

We wouldn't take poisonous and damaging psychotropic drugs for the flu. We know enough about the disease to understand it isn't worth that kind of risk. We wouldn't allow our civil rights to be taken from us for the flu. We wouldn't allow anyone to fry our brains, or even our nasal passages, to get rid of the flu.

Education makes the critical difference. That's why this book exists – to educate people about the myths of bipolar and perhaps, just perhaps, save some people – people like the 26 case studies that follow – from a lifetime of chemical dependence and patronising psychobabble, as well as symptoms of a cure that could come straight from Dante's *Inferno*.

What allows pharmaceutical companies and psychiatrists to treat people the way they do is the commoditisation of human life and experience. To Big Pharma and Big Psychiatry, patients are consumers of a product – not people. But people are what they are, and people *suffer* Big Pharma and Big Psychiatry, just as they suffer the symptoms of disease. Knowledge and education lead to a weakened resolve to resort to psychiatry and pharmaceutical terrors, which in turn, over a slow process of time, might yet lead to a revolution in the way we think about bipolar, mental illness, and psychiatry in general.

Mary

I wanted to travel the world and so went ahead and bought a round-the-world ticket before giving away all my possessions. The day before I left Ireland I went out and spent hundreds of pounds on chocolate to take to the children in Africa. I hadn't thought how I was going to get it there without it melting beforehand. I decided my first stop was going to be Greece, because I wanted to read the *Book of Revelations* where it was written.

My mania always has a very spiritual side to it.

I travelled twelve hours by ferry from Athens to Pathos Island to the Monastery of Saint John the Baptist, where I sat and read the whole book. I was ecstatic at that stage, totally and utterly happy beyond belief at this accomplishment. Within days of getting to Patmos I felt like I knew everyone. My manic episode had well and truly reached its zenith. I was so happy, full of love and seemed to connect with everyone. I went out all night and danced until dawn, drinking water. I wasn't eating anything at this point and barely sleeping.

Days later I was arrested for running around naked. I was hand-cuffed and thrown into a filthy cell, and eventually moved to a stinking hospital. It was my first psychiatric admission. I was terrified. All I had was the dress I had been wearing and a Bible. The days that followed were spent in utter confusion. I was fed fish with their heads and tails on and stale bread. Against my will, I was held down and injected twice a day with the drug Largactil, which made me feel trapped and claustrophobic, and had the unpleasant side-effect of making me photosensitive. My only means of communication with my fellow patients was through accepting cigarettes. Eventually, a representative from the Irish Embassy came to my rescue and sorted out my travel arrangements back to Ireland.

As soon as I got back to Ireland, my body went into a strange state. I now know it to be a reaction to the antipsychotic medication I had been receiving in Greece, but initially I had no idea what was happening to me. I became extremely restless and felt as if I had ants under my skin. I couldn't stand or sit. No position felt comfortable. It was horrendous. At this point, I still didn't have a diagnosis, so I had no idea what was happening. I made my way to the Accident and Emergency department at my local hospital only to be told that no beds were available, so they sent me home. This happened four days in a row until they eventually found a bed. A day later, I was diagnosed with bipolar disorder.

Nothing prepares you for your own diagnosis. The doctor was quite cavalier. He looked at my chart and said "It's obvious what's going on here – your father has bipolar disorder and you have it too," before walking off. I will never forget the fear that went through me. A day later, I had my first encounter with the psychiatrist. He told me that my judgement had been impaired since birth and that after eight to fifteen years on Lithium I would be fine. I was horrified. I felt that all the achievements in my life had been undermined. I felt that I was staring at an impossible future. I would be angry, violent and dependent, just like my father. It was a frightening scenario. Because of my father's condition, I thought I understood bipolar disorder. I read voraciously on the condition. And yet when I was diagnosed myself, none of this helped. I felt abject terror and there was no guidance from anywhere. You are given a label that separates you from humanity and then set adrift.

The battle with medication began. Within a couple of months on Lithium I was a complete vegetable. I gained two stone and spent my days watching quiz programmes on television, incapable of doing anything else. I was totally and utterly miserable. The doctors asked me to give it more time. Lithium is the miracle drug for eighty per cent of sufferers. That leaves twenty per cent of us who are not so lucky. I gave it nine months. My life was in a shambles. I flushed it down the toilet and moved to Dublin to stay with my brother. A terrible bout of depression ensued, where I worried for my life. I felt utterly wretched, prompting me to ask my brother to take me to the hospital.

Everybody feels the blues. Everybody experiences grief. Everybody cries. So what is bipolar depression really like? In my experience it has a pattern. It is a slow withdrawal from life. A loss of interest in the everydayness of things which progresses to full-scale isolation in one's mind. You can be in the proverbial crowded room and still feel disconnected to everybody. There is a serious drain of energy, which no amount of sleep seems to redress. One's inner thought patterns become flooded with negative messages. You feel a failure – no matter what you've achieved in life. These thoughts are overwhelming and constant. You lose all self-respect and your self-grooming goes awry too. Otherwise capable people are reduced to shadows of themselves and even minor tasks, like housework, can cause panic in a person. If you are of a spiritual bent, this state may bring terror of hell or feeling too sinful for God ever to forgive you. You battle isolation from stigma and ignorance. Suicidal depression kicks in. You feel useless and worthless. Depression is a response to stress and pressure. To survive, you must switch off and go to a place of refuge. All is bleak.

Life in a psychiatric ward is never dull. Initially I was quite frightened, but like anything in life, once you've experienced something you normalise it. Medication time brought everyone together. Everyone followed the 'zombie cart', got their fix and talked about their side-effects. These could often be more uncomfortable than anything your condition was throwing at you. The effect is like wearing a chemical straightjacket. Your limbs are paralysed and your speech is impaired. Many notions about the psychiatrically ill come from perceptions of people on these drugs. It all creates fear and a lack of understanding. It is not the disorder that causes these reactions – it is the treatment. To this day, I shudder at the lack of support there was for this process. I once requested an appointment to see a psychologist. That was twenty years ago and I am still waiting.

But to get to the root of the whole situation, I have to go back in time. My childhood had been fractious and my figuring out of life was done without support. Time wasn't wasted on little worries in our house. I had to learn to keep things to myself. I started secondary school when I was twelve and had to listen to daily taunts telling me how ugly and fat I was. I was a *freak* because I had a desire to go on to third level education. This aspiration seemed an impossible dream for a rural working class girl to achieve. Always on the outside peering in. Some evenings I went with my mother after school to visit my father in hospital. We had to pass through several locked doors to get to the ward where we would find him sitting, wearing glasses with one of the lenses missing and the other cracked. Looking around, I saw men through my childish eyes, hiding from imaginary Russians under their beds. And then there was the mystique of seeing the padded cells when we were escorted out at the end of the visit. My mother was always fraught with worry. I locked myself in prayer before and after these visits, but God seemed far away in the distance from me.

I was aware from a very young age that all was not well with my father. In seventies Ireland, bipolar disorder, or manic depression as it was then called, was a big label to carry. Totally misunderstood by those around him, he sought solace in alcohol. He didn't have a lot of insight into his condition and this wreaked havoc with family life. My childhood fascination with God was born from negotiating my father's illness. You had to believe to survive. My father used to disappear for months at a time and I never knew where or why. Snippets of information came my way through listening to adult whispers and things that were said at national school. Other kids knew where my father was. They told me he was in the *madhouse*. There was only one place worse, and everybody knew that was hell.

At seventeen, I left home to go to college to study Philosophy and English Literature. I loved college life and the freedom and liberation I found in city life after a sheltered life in the countryside. I partied, made new friends, discovered new interests and fell deeply in love. My life was really on track, but just after I graduated, a tragedy struck that changed my life. My boyfriend, who was my first love, drowned in a fishing accident. I can still remember the shattering, crushed feeling when I was told the news. The man who had made me feel special and protected was dead. I just couldn't handle it because I didn't have the inner resources at the time. His mother gave me his coat. I wore it until it lost his smell. Then I wore it some more. I wandered around at night, fighting insomnia. I just wanted to follow him. This was the only time I came close to killing myself. I didn't want to die, but I couldn't bear the mental torture in my brain anymore. I began to drink to anaesthetise the pain. I wanted to drown myself and was about to do it when a man out walking found me on a bridge, and with great patience and understanding talked me down and saved my life. When you are at that point you feel everyone is better off without you. You just can't bear the thoughts in your head anymore. But I recovered after this incident and decided that a change of direction was needed in my life, so I decided to go travelling again. However, after arriving in London I went through a period of terrifying night terrors and hallucinations, but did not feel able to seek help. Debilitated by depression, I felt useless. I was twenty-one and began to realise that the physical move was not the answer; it was something inside of me that was wrong. Alcohol was still my main medication. I eventually got a job in a hotel working as a receptionist and dragged myself in every day. After six months of this existence, I decided to move again. This time I went to Amsterdam and I fell in love again – although this time it wasn't with a man, rather a fantasy.

Although I had suffered depression many times, I had never before experienced mania that was this extreme. It started off with a feeling of inordinate wellbeing. I stopped drinking and smoking. I walked around feeling totally happy. I believed myself to be in love, but it was no ordinary love. We were Genesis 2, the new Adam and Eve. We were going to create a New World Order. God was positivity and light. There was a gospel of cool and I had been given the mission to bring the message to Ireland. These were the thoughts in my head, totally high but convinced of the truth of my fantasy. I walked around barefoot in all weathers and danced and partied every night, drinking nothing except water. I slept wherever I was offered a bed.

The whole universe becomes unbearably beautiful. Sights and sounds and music become amplified and I can spend hours gazing at a grain of dirt and find it truly beautiful. Everything becomes dreamlike and surreal. My thoughts race through my brain at frightening speed. I recall believing that I was on a giant chessboard, playing chess with human figures. Weightlessness and feelings of actually becoming part of my surroundings (like if I lean against a rock, I will become part of it) feature regularly in my thoughts. Water is another fascination. Walking into water, I feel no separation between the water and myself. The next stage is the psychotic stage where I enter a dream world and see hallucinations and have delusions. Although I am faintly aware of reality, the reality I am seeing is totally different to those watching me. At this stage I am not sleeping or eating. I feel linked to the whole universe in a very special and spiritual way.

I eventually settled down, but the mania was followed with a depressive episode again. As Isaac Newton discovered, what goes up must come down – and I did with a bang. It was indescribably dark and I was in pain, with my mental torture constant and unabating. I took to my bed and wondered if I would ever see the world outside my window ever again. But thankfully, I survived yet again to tell the tale. Then, after a decade of battling periods of depression and mania, I reached a point of stability and grasped this chance to move to England to start a new life. I left with the princely sum of £80 in my pocket. Four months later I had a permanent job and I bought my first house. These are halcyon days in my memory. For the next two years, I taught in one of the toughest schools in Essex and rose to the challenge. I took my tablets every day and enjoyed a normal existence. It is one of the happiest periods of my troubled life. I was strong, independent and fully functioning.

I had seen a homeopath before I left Ireland and she had really helped me. By now, although I was well I realised that I was taking chemicals into my body every day that were toxic in the long term. I wanted to find a cure and then help others if I could. I enrolled in the College of Practical Homeopathy and began to study on a part-time basis. Homoeopathy is a gentle energy medicine that is over 200 years old. It operates by using the Law of Similars or treating like with like. I started to slowly cut back on medication under the auspices of the homeopath. It was a two-year process, but eventually I was drug free and fine for a period of about six months. Then disaster struck. I was on holiday in Ireland visiting my family when I had another manic episode. This time I went high quickly and without warning. In the past it had taken months to go up and months to come down. This time it was a matter of hours. At first, I became really quiet and uncommunicative. My family thought I was depressed, by which time they alerted psychiatric services that I was exhibiting strange behaviour. It took six nurses to restrain me because in my deluded state I thought I was made of dough and that the nurses were trying to get me into an oven to bake me. I remember the terror, because this was absolutely real to me at that time. I soldiered on through night terrors and hallucinations. The medication I had taken in the past was no longer effective. The search was on for a new combination. This time, Sodium Valproate was prescribed.

I gained three stone within a couple of months, was utterly miserable and my life had descended into total chaos. I am a strong, capable person when well, but life had become unmanageable. Bills mounted up, relationships were in turmoil and I couldn't cope with the outside world. If I had won the lottery during this time I still wouldn't have been able to leave the couch. I wasn't able to work so I had to sell my house in England and ended up living with my parents again, existing on disability payments.

Like everyone, I was brought up to believe doctors know best. Twelve years of coping with mental illness have led me to believe that this is not necessarily true – especially with the way they perceive mental disorder. In the main, doctors are trained to accept a medical model of illness, which has the belief that all disorders are chemical in nature. Address the chemical imbalance, address the disorder, which in other words means that once they have the patient chemically balanced they see their job as done. While drug therapy has a role to play, doctors need a wider vision to work from. But yet we are asked to continue to trust in a health system that refuses to see us as individuals, but would rather perceive us as the label they have for a condition we suffer from. Every time I go for a check-up, I am seen by a different psychiatrist, who has never read my file beforehand, so I have to go over my case – which is a complete waste of time. I have lost faith in my GP too, because his answer to bipolar is that I should accept that I am handicapped.

There are times when I still feel useless and worthless. I have no place among my people. They reject me every time I seek help. I join committees and I helped to set up a support group. I am vocal about my illness, happy to be the mad woman in the village, hoping to make it easier for others. But all I feel is rejection. I have no husband, no children. I am not part of the infrastructure. I tried to get work in my local school and submitted a job application but they never contacted me. Eventually I got some work teaching English to foreign nationals. There was a silent acknowledgement between us that only the disenfranchised understand. A local bigot castigates me for doing this work whenever we meet. Once I walked into the local supermarket and was asked by the shop assistant, "Are you right yet? You've been in hospital enough times." Then there are those who stop me on the street and assure me of their prayers. Some enquire as to what I do all day. I mostly get described as poor Mary or *that one* with bipolar.

What, in the end, is a mental illness? For me, bipolar is a journey of the soul. It is the response of the human organism to stress and pressure. To survive, the organism must switch off in the form of depression to survive or fly into elation. Both are places of refuge. Though it has been difficult at times, I wouldn't swap my life for any other. Why? Because into all existence, rain falls. But oh, the sunshine! I have experienced the full gamut of emotion. I have been entrenched in the pit of despair, but I have also experienced Eden. Maybe the price was high; maybe I tread too near the Gods at times – but what a capacity it brings. You view the whole of humanity with compassion and love.

Last winter was my first time not to become depressed in nearly twenty years. It is an unbelievable feeling. I am grateful beyond belief. Summertime began yesterday. No more gloom. I am finally in recovery. I will have minor blips from time to time but in the main I am over the worst. I feel positive and well. And though much psychological damage was done in my teenage years, I have come to feel attractive and strong in my character. I may not be a supermodel, but

I will do! Health is the greatest gift that life has to offer and I have an amazing capacity for living when I am well. I love to party and to dance. I drink in moderation now. Balance in all things is the way to stay healthy.

Consultants are not open to this knowledge but are getting frustrated because patients are beginning to question their treatment. The internet throws up the lists of side-effects for every drug so people, power is slowly creeping into the system, with service users being savvier about their condition than ever before. Families in Ireland are generally insensitive with the way they deal with a child or sibling who has a mental illness, but I feel emotions like anger, sadness and pain must be expressed, no matter how uncomfortable the family is with the truth.

For all its highs and lows, my life has been an incredible journey. I feel I have enough experience to comment on the services in Ireland when I say the mentally ill are still the untouchables of Irish society. In general they are the forgotten in any health budget. As a rule, they have no voice. They are too consumed with pain to be part of the decision-making process in their lives. They are not a powerful lobby in the corridors of power. Simply, no one really gives a damn about mental health. Mentally ill people are not politically active, meaning very few vote. Most people with a diagnosis of mental health eke out meagre existences on disability allowances.

I am now in remission and hopefully on the road to permanent recovery. I know I cannot say that I will not have times of illness, but I also believe that no employee in any sphere can give that assurance. Will I ever be able to say, openly, that I need a week off for a little fine-tuning – just like normal people who get the flu? I feel calm and at peace with what I've got in life. There is no need to fear reality anymore. I'm giving it a real go. For all it's worth, I feel the inner maelstrom has subsided.

I am positive about the future. These days I'm in the forgiveness business. Love is all about letting go. I still travel, and last year I went to Rome. I stood in the Sistine Chapel and was moved to tears by the beauty of its ceiling. The power of imagination went right to my head. But I was stable this time. Totally lucid – and in that state of stability, felt release knowing that beauty, as I have seen in my imaginings, actually exists – and with this came a profound sense of peace.

Adam

My unquiet mind is always busy – it never stops. During my teenage years I struggled with girls and did not lose my virginity until my mid-twenties. I viewed myself as an outsider and inwardly didn't understand why others around me couldn't understand the discrepancy between their perceptions of me and how I felt about myself. At one point, I thought heterosexual love had eluded me and toyed with the idea that I might be gay, but after a while it became clear I wasn't attracted to men. Then I met a girl who I placed on a pedestal. She was perfect and someone I thought would gain my parents' approval. But they disliked her personality and felt she lacked ambition because she didn't want to go to university, so our relationship petered out. Although I had a few brief affairs afterwards, it was only recently that I met a lovely girl on an internet dating site. We have really formed a tight bond together. I have been totally honest with her about my bipolar because I didn't want any secrets to come between us, which she appreciates.

My parents were decent working class people who had aspirations for their children. We have always got on well together but at the same time there was a detachment between us. Our communications and interactions were cordial but bordered on aloof. When I was young there were no hugs or kisses and I never confided my fears, hopes or secrets with them. But nevertheless they were kind parents and God knows they have rescued me from tricky situations dozens of times over the years. My mother was the worst for having set ideas on politics and religion but my father too was pretty conservative. They were forthright in their views on what they saw as best for me and this started when I was sent away to boarding school. This later extended to university, before moving their ideals onto me having the perfect relationship, the perfect career, the perfect home and car and the perfect wife and children. The list was endless. If I didn't get an *A* in my exams I felt I would not be loved – so there was an ongoing desire to achieve success for them.

I attended university, studying Mathematical Science. There I mingled with people from privileged backgrounds and although I made friends, I recognised I was unable to interact freely or feel at ease. I would spend hours by myself in my room, analysing people's reactions to what I had said in everyday conversations. Around this time I went through an experimental phase with drugs – mainly cannabis, but I also took cocaine from time to time.

During my third year at university, the stress of the exams and fear of failure resulted in me sinking into a deep depression. I couldn't get out of bed and was unable to do anything on a meaningful level. I couldn't stand people around me and just stayed in bed for days on end. I went to my GP, who prescribed Prozac. I also attended some counselling at the practice, but there was no exploration by my GP as to what might have caused the depression. The Prozac took time to work but eventually my mood lifted. It felt like the sky cleared and removed its dark clouds – making me suddenly become sociable, talkative and confident. The new *me* had come out of its shell. This went on for weeks before my behaviour at a party became so euphoric, it was described later as aggressive – but I was on a high and loved it.

Shortly after finishing my degree, I decided to take a break, and on a whim took a job as a tour guide in Spain. I remember travelling by train to Gatwick airport and feeling totally uncomfortable about other passengers around me. I didn't want to meet their gaze and was terrified that someone would talk to me. It was like being trapped in a cage with a wild animal, having to keep still, knowing the slightest movement could prompt the beast to pounce. After a few days I became acutely aware that there had been a massive shift in my mood. I was no longer confident – no longer articulate. The new job was horrendous. I wasn't able to cope with the pressure of being around people all the time and after six months I resigned and returned home. My parents were concerned about me and encouraged me to seek medical attention. More or less the same story ensued again. I received a sympathetic ear from the doctor along with another prescription of Prozac, and another referral to see the practice counsellor.

I was angry with myself and felt a failure. My parents were not so much angry as disappointed when I told them I didn't want to pursue a career in mathematics or accountancy – as I had developed a completed aversion towards figures and calculations. I knew this meant not fulfilling their aspirations. They had invested money and hope into my success, but here I was in my early twenties, back living with them, without a job or money. I felt like a dependant teenager, receiving financial support in the form of weekly pocket money until my benefits were sorted out, making me cringe every time it was handed to me.

A couple of months later I started a new low-key administrative job in a neighbouring town. It felt good to go outdoors again after several months lying in a darkened room, motionless while staring at the wall, wishing for something to happen. After a few weeks into the new job I became aware that my mood was buoyant again and felt relief when I was able to be sociable, confident and articulate with colleagues. But although I didn't want to acknowledge it, I had a gut feeling that something was terribly wrong. I even began going out for drinks and meals with new friends. Everything felt good – both personally and professionally. Admittedly, I was curt at times to colleagues, but they jokingly teased me about the intellectual vanity in my character. Then the bleakest depression I ever experienced descended upon me like a kite, falling to the ground in a vengeful storm. The depression was so bad I could see no way through the mire of darkness, and I ended up taking a large overdose of Paracetamol, resulting in hospitalisation. The hospital did not deem me a danger to myself. What I had done was considered to be a cry for help. I was discharged back to my doctor and this time was prescribed different antidepressants. The prospect of returning to work filled me with dread. The atmosphere at home was tense. I couldn't turn to my parents and tell them how I was feeling. I knew they must have felt powerless – helpless in fact. What was taking place was alien to them. They remained supportive, but none of us all were able to express our feelings to one another.

A year later I started yet again another administrative job. My overdose was cast aside and no longer mentioned, but by now my mood was lifting again at an alarming rate. I decided to move into a shared house. The newfound freedom felt good. I began to smoke cannabis again. It relaxed me a little but it didn't mask my high spirits because my manager called me into the office and asked me outright if I was on drugs – such was the extent of my wayward and relentlessly buoyant behaviour. I became upset at his audacity in challenging me like that and a terse argument resulted in me losing my job. I wasn't too upset though because I wasn't short of money, having recently acquired three credit cards with a collective spending limit of £12,000.

I decided to return to Spain for a holiday to catch up with old friends from the tour company. Upon arrival I checked into a five-star hotel and generously entertained my friends with meals and drinks. When I flew back home I was still on a high with a cavalier disregard for everyone around me. I stayed with my parents for a while but soon got bored. They challenged me about the source of my money, but I lied. I found their company monotonous and needed stimulation – so I booked another holiday, this time to Slovenia. My mother offered to take me to the airport and during the journey challenged me again on my behaviour and financial means but I remember responding: "I'm having a good time, why should I care?" Looking back now I fully see how I was completely self-absorbed. I had no life plan. I lived for the moment and although my debts were mounting, I didn't care. After returning from Slovenia I went back to live at home again and getting another job seemed to come with the package. I ticked by for a few months by managing to lie to my parents and creditors. Then the debt collection agencies began to call at home. My parents were mortified, but I managed to bluff my way out of the situation by pacifying the *vultures* by giving them a little money. But in the long run there was no escaping my debts, and this made me deeply demoralised. I had coped with failing my parents, coped with multiple ruined jobs, coped with still living at home in my early thirties, coped with failed relationships, coped with always having felt different – being an outsider – and now I was a failure with mounting debts to overcome and it felt too much to resolve. One summer weekend, during a visit to a friend in Oxford, we drank heavily and for some inexplicable reason I ended up alone by the river. It was a sunny evening as I sat by the riverbank enviously watching tourists, young couples in love and parents playing with their children, and I imagined their happiness. My attention then became transfixed on the water. It looked so inviting that I spent two hours wishing I could slip in and end my misery. A dog-walker approached and met my gaze, making me realise that he must have known my secret. I looked around and saw him peering back in my direction as he hovered with his dog on the grass. In retrospect, I know that he was my guardian angel, because shortly afterwards I got up and went back to my friend's house. My suicidal thoughts were foiled but in the days that followed my depression increased, leaving me bedridden for weeks with angst and despair. I ended up being hospitalised and although my initial assessment upon admission mentioned 'bipolar', I wasn't given an official diagnosis for another year.

Returning home from hospital meant feeling more of a burden to my parents than ever before. The customary new job followed, with new faces in a fresh environment but it was the same old story of isolation, feelings of inadequacy and not belonging – followed by a desire to hide way from everyone. My parents kindly paid off my debts and also arranged for me to see a private counsellor, but I found this difficult and I was guarded in my sessions. However, I eventually began to feel better – but it didn't last long. Within six months my moods elevated once more. I remember going out to lunch one day with a friend. My voice became so loud in the restaurant that I was overheard making derogatory remarks about our employer within earshot of fellow diners, which resulted in word getting back to my boss, who sacked me immediately. I didn't care because I had just conned my way into getting another £10,000 loan from the bank in order to set up my own modelling agency. It was just another idiotic idea without any logical explanation. I didn't have an interest in fashion, nor any background or experience in the field, but I researched business plans on the internet for three days non-stop without eating or sleeping. I tricked my way into arranging a business meeting with executives in London and attempted to get them to go along with my scam. At the meeting I espoused a plethora of ideas with haste. Excitement made my voice grow louder as I paced up and down while doing a presentation from my laptop. Proverbially speaking, I was foaming at the mouth by the end of my speech but within half an hour my high-spirited mood had begun to plummet with a vengeance. I became so overcome by what can only be described as a tidal wave of emotion that I cried uncontrollably before walking into a department store and asking an assistant to call an ambulance.

Hospital was absolute hell. I was given drug after drug to stabilise my mood. I felt disorientated and couldn't bear the thoughts of seeing my family. Finally, I was officially diagnosed with bipolar disorder and given Diazepam to calm me down. My journey to diagnosis took a full six years and by this time had amounted to multiple depressive episodes followed by periods of mania. I often imagine a graph in my head that charts my moods during these lost years. It's a perfectly aligned graph, with lines going up and down – up and down – up and down – into a design that has perfect waves, capable of placing someone into a hypnotic hold. After I left hospital I was discharged into the care of my local community mental health team. I was placed on Lithium the following year and I still remain on this today, along with antipsychotics and sleeping tablets. This combination works for me and prevents me from relapsing.

Life is good at present but it would be better if I could get a grasp of my drinking. This is easier said than done. When I'm challenged to do something about it, I go into denial, claiming that my consumption isn't a problem. But I know it is really, especially at weekends, making me unable to work five days a week because I need every Monday and Tuesday off to recover from my excesses. I also justify it by saying that I look after my health by not smoking, by exercising and eating healthily. But the truth is that I drink because it takes the edge off the intensity of my feelings. With a drink in my hand, I find I am at my funniest and tell the wittiest anecdotes.

What does the future hold? Although I am still living with my parents I manage to live a fairly independent life. I have a regular group of friends and never seem short of things to do. My new job is with a mental health advocacy charity, where I help other service-users sort out difficulties by reassuring them that bipolar is a word, not a sentence. The advocacy service tells people that with accurate diagnosis and treatment it is possible to have a good quality of life. We let people know they are in control by enabling them to make informed choices, including the likely outcomes if they don't seek medical treatment – practical support along with visiting a GP – and explaining the pathway into community mental health services. Knowledge about bipolar is real power, so we provide information about support groups, such as the *Bipolar Foundation*. We also help people to look at practical issues, such as financial management if someone is in a manic episode and see what support is available for family members or carers. If there is an issue with medication, as there was for me when I was switched from Sodium Valproate to Lithium, we support clients in approaching their consultant for a review, in the hope of changing to another medication with positive results.

I feel lucky that I haven't relapsed in a long time and attribute this to my awareness of my moods, knowing I must intervene and seek help the moment I notice a change. Then there is Laura, with whom I am hoping for a future. She has been great and I feel we have a real connection. She has just finished reading my favourite book on bipolar, *An Unquiet Mind* by Kay Redfield Jamison. Unless you have experienced the highs and low of bipolar disorder, you can never truly understand its darkness, confusion or the frightening ordeal that comes as part of the condition. But this book, which was written by a psychologist with bipolar, greatly increases understanding for family and friends of someone with the condition. Laura said she found it was an eye-opening read and it helped her to realise how confusing it is for someone with bipolar – whose reality is out of sync with the rest of the world. It would be great to get married one day and have kids. These were probably things I should have done fifteen or twenty years ago, but I would still like to do them now, rather than never. Right now, I'm feeling good about my life and am determined not to let anyone get in the way of my happiness again. Wish me luck!

When I'm unwell – I am:

1. Stressed
2. Fearful
3. Selfish, with no regard for others
4. Exhausted
5. Either quiet or over-talkative
6. Tearful
7. Over-analytical about what people say
8. Distrusting
9. Incapable of taking care of myself or paying bills
10. Chaotic

Ian

Isobel

I have lived with bipolar for almost ten years now. In the lead-up to an episode I can't sleep for a couple of nights and get overactive. Then it's like a light switch goes off and I am suddenly completely delusional.

I have always had a bit of a fetish for deserts. This stems back to my childhood when I loved to walk barefoot across the sand on the beach, feeling its soft, warm and silky touch. Episodes of mania rekindle these feelings but in a paranoid, bizarre and disturbing way. I read fervently about the Sahara, Arabian and Kalahari, all the great deserts of the world, and when unwell I am convinced that a supreme force conspires with nature to cover the entire earth with sand, over-ruling soil and making it redundant in the process. A programme on television about sandstorms reinforced my belief even further. I saw how powerful sand was in those storms and decided that soil could never be like that. It was too lazy to move and so the time had come for it to suffer because of its ineptitude. The reality of my imaginings were so strong that I constantly went to the window to check if the ground has become covered in sand, like someone does when they are expecting snow in wintertime.

It's utter nonsense, but I believe it very strongly and there is no point whatsoever in anyone attempting to converse with me, as I will be terrified of everyone and everything. I always compare bipolar to a volcano erupting or a geyser that goes off every Friday at five o'clock. It feels like a natural explosion in the brain that happens every so often, just like epilepsy.

After taking antipsychotics, the whole thing winds down, for the most part within a week to three weeks. Then I'm a hundred per cent sane again for several years, before it happens again. Having had severe episodes of both mania and depression, I can assure you the disorder is real. But the amazing thing is that the last three manic episodes I had happened when I was taking a lot of medication, which included Lithium and antipsychotics. When I'm well I often ask myself, 'Why am I taking this medication?' I think treatment should be limited to the manic episodes. It just seems crazy to take these awful medications that don't work on a continuous basis. I finally understand why over sixty-five per cent of people with bipolar are non-compliant – most of them secretly.

My psychiatrist won't answer questions when I ask about reducing the medication. I have argued so much with her over the years. It is my belief that if I take a large dose of antipsychotic medication for two days during a manic episode, it will be quickly resolved. But my psychiatrist totally discounts this and refuses to discuss it. Have you ever tried to argue with a psychiatrist? It is not a pretty sight. She makes fraudulent claims about medication, insisting that I need to take it for life to ensure I control the severity of both manic and depressive episodes – otherwise I will become a degenerate. It is part of her dark fairy tale. The other part is her instruction to be a good girl, take the medication and if I go to bed early every night I won't have as many episodes. With regards to side-effects, she bluntly said "No gain without pain," before brazenly stating the worst reactions from the medication would still be much easier to tolerate than bipolar itself. But the bleak reality reveals psychiatric drugs to be an entombment, which for me consisted of persistent diarrhoea and blurred vision. It's a terrible shock when you've endured a truly horrible regimen of Lithium and antipsychotics for 'maintenance' and have breakdowns anyway. I know now that she was merely a conduit for the pharmaceutical sales representative and not a proper doctor who wanted to help. Basically, psychiatrists, under the influence of pharmaceutical companies, insist patients take these terrible drugs for years – although they have no preventative effect, even at lower doses.

Psychiatrists have come up with this really offensive suggestion that people with bipolar enjoy being manic – loving the adrenaline, drama and recklessness that invariably comes with the condition. But I think this is absolute rubbish. I don't think any person, even those who are insane, would wish such misery and dysfunction upon themselves. The truth is that we just want to be like everyone else and to live happy, uncomplicated lives, with normal feelings and emotions.

But at the moment I feel trapped and have felt like this for many years. You cannot just suddenly quit Lithium or any other antipsychotic medication, or you risk becoming very ill. I would like to get off Lithium, but it would take a year to do this gradually. I definitely advocate a critique of the treatment of bipolar. However, I believe that medication is a necessary evil, but one that should be used sparingly. I've had loads of high-quality therapy but trust me, talking about things bears no relationship to bipolar episodes. I have also found that most therapists don't have the slightest clue about bipolar and its presentation – or its consequences – the regime of medication and side-effects and the feeling of never being free from it. Support groups aren't much good either, unless people there also have bipolar.

I mainly try to keep my bipolar secret because of a bad experience I had with a former friend. We were out at dinner along with a male friend of hers. It was a nice restaurant, the food was good and we were merrily chatting about various news items and politics when, during the conversation, my friend flippantly remarked on how much she thought the Government does for crazy people – pointing at me in the process. The tone of her voice revealed superiority, indicating how she valued her sanity over mine. Her friend laughed loudly when a thwarted attempt was made to discuss what happens when people become manic. It was quite an upsetting incident and to be honest I don't want to deal with something like that again – so I keep my little *secret* to myself. Besides, bipolar is extremely hard to explain to people, so I generally don't bother. On the other side of the coin, you have to deal with psychiatric personnel – nurses and social workers – who want to treat mental patients as if they have intellectual disabilities. It sometimes feels as if they are annoyed when someone has a strong intellect and seems they would consider it much easier for themselves to have the patient on antipsychotics – effectively lobotomised – that way, you do as they ask. Given psychiatry's poor track record with bipolar and the abuses that have gone along with that, I think it would be better to treat bipolar under neurology, like epilepsy. But for now I take the medication and keep my mouth shut. But in true *Shawshank Redemption** style,

I am eyeing up my escape route and looking for a way out of this psychiatric *prison* which can easily become a way of life. Okay, it's not a real prison with bars, locks, cells or orderlies but nevertheless it feels like a *prison* where any person clasped within its grip becomes as institutionalised as any real prisoner whose freedom has been taken away.

* The Shawshank Redemption (1994) is a film, based on a Stephen King novella, about a banker who is falsely accused of a double murder. During his long stretch in prison, he comes to be admired by the other inmates for his upstanding moral code and his quietly indomitable spirit – and then he escapes and finds freedom.

Luke

When I look back now at my late teens, I see the largest hole and still feel the speed of my actions as I entered it. When I was manic, I attended parties everywhere whether I was invited or not because having a good time was all that mattered. I was continuously buzzing and rarely slept. It was no problem to keep active for three days in a row without even sitting down. Maybe the reason I neglected rest was because I knew the flip side of mania meant days just sat staring at the television with a dead feeling inside. Being depressed means having a longing for deep rest. It is so boring. You don't want to do anything. Sleep is the only thing on your mind and when you eventually go to bed, you don't want to ever get up again, spending most days just laying there dozing.

When I was younger I felt lousy about myself. I'm sure my low self-confidence led to me becoming depressed. So I drank anything up to ten pints of lager at a time to numb my feelings. Looking back now I realise that being depressed is a loss of life. The world goes on around you, but you feel you are stuck under frozen ice covering a lake. It takes tremendous strength and willpower to break through the ice to breathe again and start living.

It was hard being around the house when I was young, because my father had periods of illness in which he was verbally abusive, raising his voice and lashing out at everyone in the family – especially after he returned home from the pub. I would sit close to my mother during those times, thinking I had to protect her. By the time I was in my late teens, I was showing signs of becoming as erratic as my father. But my real periods of mania occurred from my twenties onwards, when I started smoking skunk. That really screwed my head up. I began to see things all the time – lightning in the sky, spiders everywhere, and I was always imagining that there was something wrong with my feet.

I know now that I was paranoid. One Sunday, I took the dog with me to Mass. The church was crowded when I walked up the aisle – feeling the full stare of everyone as I passed through. My little venture didn't stop there. After Mass had finished, I went over to the local pub, walked straight behind the bar, poured myself a pint of beer, took a sip and then walked out again. The barman knew my parents and didn't make a fuss. My mum was also affected by my father's aggressive outbursts – and I guess by mine as well. She, too, had periods of depression and found it hard to cope at times – but is that any wonder? I learned my lesson the hard way. The answer is to keep clean by staying away from the skunk.

We were never alive at the same time, having just missed each other by a matter of months, but that has never prevented me from feeling extraordinarily close to Aidan, my little brother who died of cot death shortly before I was born. I felt he was my guardian angel and was sure I could feel his protective presence towering over me. As a child I always worried about everyone, and this became so unbearable at times that I used to cycle up to Aidan's grave, which was in the cemetery in the next village, and sit by his graveside, praying to him for help for someone or other in our family. So close was my connection to my dead brother that whenever I drew pictures at home or in school I used to tell everyone that it was Aidan and I who drew them or I would write both our names at the bottom of the drawings.

At other times, I used to pray that my family would win the lottery. I also prayed that my dad would be kept safe as he drove home from the pub at weekends. I cried my heart out to God, asking him to never take my parents away from me. This was probably the start of my bipolar. When I was fourteen, I remember sitting with the family doctor. She said to me, "You have bipolar disorder like your mum and dad." I was shy in front of the doctor. Too shy to speak on my own and too shy to ask my mother to explain what the doctor had said. I felt embarrassed, guilty in fact that I wasn't considered normal. No one mentioned a cure, but then I remember reckoning that mad people could never be cured.

Throughout secondary school, I rode one rollercoaster after another. I moved from one group to another all the time and could never settle with any of my friends for long. One day I'd be happy – full of horseplay, full of chat – and then the next day I'd come in and wouldn't be able to speak. Teachers and fellow students used to ask me what was wrong, but I couldn't find the words to tell them how I felt. My mind was full of thoughts but the words would not come out to tell them what I was thinking. So, unable to speak, I held back my words and energy and wrapped myself up in my thoughts inside my own crazy little world of a mind.

Nothing happens fast in the world of psychiatry, so it's best not to be in a rush. Psychiatrists seem to come and go all the time. The last time I went to see my psychiatrist, I was told he was on holidays and that I would have to see a junior female doctor on his team. She was young, and knew nothing about me, started asking me lots of questions. She hardly looked at me, just sat there firing off questions while reading through the notes on my file. I cut her short and told her I had answered all these questions dozens of times before. Then I asked for a change of medication because the Lithium was giving me terrible headaches and nightmares. All she said was that she was unable to make any changes until my consultant returned, but that my request would then be considered. That was over a year ago and I am still waiting to have my prescription reduced or changed.

How can people say they are treated well by doctors when some of them reach for the prescription pad without first finding out the basics, like does a person have enough food? They don't seem to have the time to listen or to find out what is really going on. Nurses, in my experience, are little better, and should take real time out to talk to their patients. They barely say 'hello.' I witnessed it myself when I was in hospital, how they would remain in the office eighty-five per cent of the time, talking and laughing amongst themselves.

I don't like it when people call bipolar an illness. They want to give it a label. They think it explains what is wrong, but it only creates negative stereotypes. My mother always said the world would be a weird place if everyone was the same. Some people, though, are more sensitive than others – but I give everyone a chance, really. There are those that don't talk as much as others, but are gifted people in their own right. I'm sure some people have had a hard childhood and sadly will not be able to change. I'm lucky I didn't give up. My motto is why give up when you only live once? I have learned to live with bipolar. It's fine now I have it under control.

But it's hard to explain to people sometimes about bipolar when they have no experience themselves of what it feels like. My girlfriend, in this respect, was no different when we first met. I tried telling her but couldn't find the right moment. Then I stopped taking my medication and although everything was okay for a while, slowly I started to become hyperactive and knowing as I did that whenever this starts, it's usually followed by a long depression, I sought medical help. I ended up being hospitalised for a while and this helped me in the sense that a close friend of mine broke the news of my illness to her. She visited me in hospital and from that moment on she gradually came to understand what was wrong with me. It has brought us closer together and enriched our love for one another. But having to go back into hospital was horrible. As I said, I dislike psychiatrists, with psychiatric nurses in second place. They all smile – big smarmy, superficial smiles – all the time. They never listen. They never wanted to hear my side of the story. Their agenda was purely a matter of deciding on what medication to feed me and to make sure I took it.

Football is my passion. Actually, all sport is a massive part of my life. I am a huge supporter of Manchester United and follow all their matches. On my days off from the local bakery where I work I can be found in front of the television watching Sky Sports. I also love Gaelic football and soccer. I play every weekend on two different teams with friends. We practice during the week after work. I have a soccer cup final coming up soon and a Gaelic match championship as well.

Over the years, I have learned ways to escape boredom. One of these methods is to simply take out a biro and start writing down my precise thoughts at that time. I have also got into the habit of writing most days and have figured out that if I write an A4 page every day, it will add up to thousands of words over the course of a year. It's the therapeutic aspect of writing that I enjoy best, as well as a sense of achievement. Some of my mutterings are about nature, which I have always loved. I remember as a young boy lying awake early in the morning, my head filled with dread about school and the day ahead of me, when I'd hear my uncle, who lived next door, start the engine of his bread van shortly after 5am, breaking the dawn silence. After he had driven off, I would just lay there and listen to the birds singing. It was so soothing, and because of memories like this, I firmly believe that nature will always be more powerful than human beings.

My older brother returned home to visit one weekend. He is only three years older than me but left school early and moved away. We went out socialising together and got chatting over a few drinks, resulting in him breaking down and apologising for leaving me behind at home; for knowing how lonely I would be and how I would have to bear the weight of the crap and madness that went on in our dysfunctional household. He apologised for knowing that some mad doctor had put ideas into my head, at the age of thirteen, that I too was becoming bipolar like my father, without ever stopping and thinking for a second about the enormous pressure this would put on my shoulders; how frightened of the future it made me – how scared of my own shadow I became. But I've managed happiness at last,

I think, and haven't touched alcohol or smoked skunk in a long time. Thank God I have plenty of life in my body and that I enjoy sport so much. I hope we win the championship this year. I'm on my way now into town to meet my girlfriend with *Fernando* blasting in my earplugs………*There was something in the air that night, the stars were bright, Fernando. There were shinning there for you and me, for liberty, Fernando.* ……

Ha Ha Ha!

Words that define living with bipolar:

1. Denial
2. Rollercoaster
3. Caution
4. Awareness
5. Stigma
6. Truthfulness
7. Disarray
8. Humorous
9. Maturity
10. Acceptance

Catherine

Olivia

In my mind, my ideal car is parked outside my house. Its silver shade sparkles in the sunlight. It has luscious leather seats, with an immaculately valeted interior, and is complemented with a scented air-freshener smelling of wild summer berries. Parked next to it is another car, identical in colour and design, but this second car is covered in bumps and although it can still be driven, its wrecked framework renders it insufficiently roadworthy. I now imagine these two cars as people and see how my life is comparable to both of them. The first car is respected and bears all the signs and fragrances of a good life. I was this person once. I wasn't born with bipolar. My life is the result of emotional pain, and is like the second car, whose engine has become a wreck in need of repair, through neglect and bad motoring.

I had a happy childhood until my parents divorced when I was six, but shortly afterwards my life began to slope into a downward spiral. My brother and I went to live with our mother, who by any standards wasn't the most organised of people. I know there isn't a manual for raising children, because if there was my mother would have failed miserably in understanding its text. But the irony of the situation was that she was a teacher, so to the outside world we appeared to be a happy, middle-class family – but behind closed doors, a different story emerged. My mother's new partner came to live with us, resulting in frequent beatings when he was grumpy or drunk, or simply felt like thumping one of us.

We had to live with looking unkempt, never having pocket money or packed lunches and more often than not we were hungry and made to wear clothes that were too small. We made the perfect case for Social Services' intervention, yet we went unnoticed. Whether this unhappy period of my life was a trigger for my bipolar, I cannot say – but I do know something, however, that definitely was linked to it. It was a beautiful summer's day and I was sitting in my grandmother's back garden. I was thirteen at the time and there were around ten of us there preparing a barbeque. Suddenly I saw my cousin, who was in his early twenties, looking at my chest and almost at the same time I got an almighty flashback to when I was five years of age. It was like someone had walked into a dark room, switched the light on and then switched it off before walking out again. But in the brief moment that the light was turned on I remembered him sexually abusing me, distinctively recalling the images, accompanied by the excruciating physical pain of his penetration. Temporarily frozen by this realisation, the adrenaline flowed through my body, allowing me to escape from the situation by running indoors and begging my mother to take me home until she succumbed to my request.

My behaviour at home and at school deteriorated in the months that followed the flashback. I started smoking and drinking and did things with boys in the back of cars that a Catholic girl should never have done. At the same time, I developed a phobia of social situations – but this only applied when I was sober, so alcohol became the answer to help get me through the day. Every Friday, I took my mother's debit card and stole £60. This bought alcohol and cigarettes to get me through the week, but I also used some of the money in pubs and clubs, lying to my mother that I was staying with friends when the truth was I usually sought out men and spent the night with them.

Although my drinking and sexual activities continued for the next couple of years, I rather amazingly passed my A-levels and got a place at university. But the real drama was only beginning as the mania began to emerge more and more. I felt the need to be accepted, to mingle with the group, seeing my role as the class clown. At university I wanted everyone to like me, while I masked what was really happening in my head. I got a great buzz out of spending money and by the time I reached eighteen I had spent in the region of £15,000 which I'd obtained through student loans. Most of the money was spent on unnecessary rubbish like electronic gadgetry and amounted to debts, which I still owe to the present day.

I smoked cannabis daily, which gave me the false impression that life was full of fun without ever having to worry about facing a future that held responsibility. So it was all about living in the moment, having fun but at the same time being trapped in a maze of confusion with a million thoughts racing around in my head. On the one hand I didn't care about my life, yet on the other I constantly worried about being a failure.

Some people say that the dole queue is full of intellectuals, and I joined its ranks after dropping out of university before sitting my final exams. Whilst I've had several jobs over the years – ranging from working in pubs, shops, a building society and secretarial work – these never managed to last for longer than a couple of weeks because of the enduring phobia I felt by being around people, particularly men. At work, when any man spoke to me I couldn't bear to look him in the face, but after work when my female friends and I joined colleagues in a bar for drinks this would change. Aided by alcohol, my inhibitions would disappear and by the end of the night I had no qualms about going back to some man's place and having unprotected sex. Basically, I had become an unpaid prostitute.

Depression has lurked at the back of my head since my early teenage years and, with hindsight, my cousin abusing me was a contributing factor. I remember my mother taking me to a doctor and requesting that I be put on Prozac, which was her idea of motherly care. But I also believe the reason that depression never leaves me is because I have craved one thing all my life – love. Even to the present day, during moments when I feel my moods are stabilising, depression always comes back full force and takes the wind out of my sails. I have always said I can handle mania much better than depression. It's the deadness, the apathy, the hopelessness and loneliness that I cannot tolerate.

My first major depressive episode occurred in my early twenties during a relationship with someone I met in the pub one night. He controlled all my money, leaving me with nothing to pay my bills, which resulted in me getting evicted from my flat. I took an overdose and spent several months in a psychiatric hospital. There the psychiatrists debated what was wrong with me, but an analysis of my bizarre behaviour since adolescence, risky sexual practices, mood swings, alcohol and drug misuse as well as my overdose persuaded them to diagnose me with bipolar. While in hospital, I felt like I had no control over any aspect of my life, but although I felt apathetic and demoralised, manic thoughts continued to race through my mind. This contradiction made it feel like I was running along a corridor that never ended, yet my body couldn't move – leaving me bed-ridden for what seemed like an eternity.

I have been on so many medications since I was first diagnosed that I struggle to remember them all. But the one that left a particularly bad feeling behind was Amisulpride, because to my horror, my breasts filled with milk. It was just after having a termination after one of my one-night conquests and the horror of lactating was very traumatic. I was then switched to Sertaline, but this gave me anxiety so terrible that I became suicidal. I was in such a state that my mother, who usually preferred to stay in the background, insisted on coming to stay with me until a hospital bed became available. Once in hospital, I was switched to Quetiapine, which made me sleep up to eighteen hours a day. During the brief spells I was awake, I felt horribly depressed and once home I could never leave the house. This went on for several months until my psychiatrist switched my medication to Lithium, which I remain on to the present day. Some people see Lithium as a cure for bipolar, but I don't see it as being the entire answer. The only good thing about it is that it stabilised my mood swings and enabled me to seek counselling. It was during these therapy sessions that I realised that I needed to reclaim control over my life – relationships, sex life and finances. My counsellor taught me to stand up for myself and to stop worrying about other people's opinion of me. I remember walking out of the clinic at the end of a session holding my head high for the first time in ages. I call it my *light bulb moment*, because I now recognise that it was my head telling me that life was going to change – and it did, because shortly afterwards I met a wonderful man and fell in love, not lust, for the first time in my life. Shortly afterwards, I got a job in a gardening centre, which I love. There is something humbling about working with plants and shrubs and watching them grow a little more each day.

My new outlook on life has helped me to accept that life isn't about getting discharged from doctors I consider conceited, proving I can live perfectly well without them. The important things are keeping well, being happy and figuring out what you want from life before it's too late. I don't want to envisage taking medication for the rest of my life, but if it is the difference between being stable and unwell then I have no other option but to take it as long as there is a need.

My words of advice for someone newly diagnosed are to be patient and try and accept the condition for what it is – and not to consider it a life sentence. Bipolar is only a hindrance if you let it hinder you. Listen to the advice of mental health professionals but keep an open mind and educate yourself as well. Try a support group if you feel up to it and never resign yourself to a life of instability. Finally, please don't be ashamed of having bipolar.

I hate the way bipolar is portrayed on television. I cringe at the storylines in *Eastenders* and *Casualty*. I think people see bipolar as an excuse to be lazy and not work, or as scary, or perhaps as something that is contagious. Bipolar seems to be a celebrity buzzword and this really irritates me. You read of actors and singers checking into the *Priory* as if it was a luxurious hotel. They then emerge five days later, regaling interviewers with stories of their breakdown as if it were some sumptuous meal, accompanied with a side-order of bipolar. Then they go off to Marbella for a holiday, to rest and recover. A few weeks later the whole bipolar thing is completely forgotten. Well, I'm afraid it doesn't work like that in the real world because it just doesn't go away by itself – it comes and goes and even when it disappears for a while, it's still present, lurking in the background, ready to pounce upon its prey when it spots a moment of vulnerability.

I want my future to be about happiness. I want it to be a future where I can enjoy my life with my wonderful partner and our not-so-wonderful two cats that get up every morning at 4 o'clock and demand our attention. I am finally building up enough courage to take driving lessons because I still want to own my ideal car. I want to look out of the window and see my silver beauty parked on the driveway, ready to whisk me off on journeys both short and long. It will give me the freedom I need and in return will be treated with great care and respect. I will clean and polish it, making sure that a scratch never rests for long on its surface. It will never run of petrol or oil and will become a reflection of myself, both inside and out – radiating satisfaction because it will be the happiest car ever.

Nathan

Poisoning the body and expecting the mind to heal is the height of insanity: "Mind and body do not act upon each other, because they are not other, they are one."

Will Durant

The church bell rang five times. I was awake for the last four as well. It was one of those nights when my mind felt like it was being torched by fire as the mania took hold. The dormitory in the psychiatric ward didn't help, with patients shouting and staff coming in every fifteen minutes to tick the boxes on the observation forms. If you moved you were ticked off as alive, that was the only thing that mattered; if you were alive, they had succeeded.

Life was good before my breakdown. The money kept rolling in and I became pretty good at spending it. I wanted to go on holiday to somewhere warm. A travel agent suggested Rio de Janeiro, making me like the idea so much that I instantly booked it without consulting my wife or considering that our children were still in the middle of the school term. But my wife eventually warmed to the idea and smoothed things over at school. We had to travel from Manchester to Heathrow for the flight and I figured out that because there were six of us, I should buy a brand new Volkswagen Sharan for £25,000 to get us there, without a moment's thought about its cost. But my life started to change after we got back, and within eighteen months it had gone from riches to rags. It began with depression, for which I was prescribed antidepressants. But antidepressants are deceptive. After four months on them everybody, including me, thought I was getting better, but in actual fact I had begun to go high. I embraced the stock market like never before, dabbling in share dealing, as well as accepting every credit card offered to me in the era of abundant credit. The stock market is a glorified type of gambling with a strange air of the unknown about it, in the sense that when you're making money, you can't understand why, and equally when you're losing, you can't understand that either. But lose it I did, and my comfortable life was replaced with a mountain of debt. My wife found out about my £90,000 credit card debts accidentally. She feared we would be made homeless. I was manic at the time, living in a bizarre world, often disappearing for days without even mentioning I was going out. She didn't think this was good for the children's welfare and asked me to leave. After borrowing money from my brother for the trip, I decided to go to Spain and stay with friends for a while.

On my way to the airport, I got a call from my psychiatrist who said he wanted to see me as he was concerned about my behaviour. I told him I was fine and didn't want to see him. His insistence was to no avail. The sense of freedom as I travelled to Spain was amazing because no-one knew where I was and the weather was great. When I ran out of money, I came back to England to face the music. I had no money left, so I rang my brother from the airport and asked him for a lift and a place to stay. On the way to his flat, he said the GP had written me a prescription for sleeping tablets and that we needed to pick it up *en route*. When we got to the surgery, we were told the chemist had the prescription. When we got to the chemist they said they didn't have that type of medication and that we'd have to go the hospital pharmacy to collect it. On the way to the hospital, I realised I had been tricked but decided to go along with it. I was met by the Senior House officer, who looked like a Vulcan from *Star Trek*. She led me to a room where the door shut behind us with a thud. I noticed there was no handle on the inside. She then told me she had a few questions she needed answering:

Did I hear voices? No.

When I read a book did I think it was written just for me? No.

When I watched television were there hidden messages for me? No.

Then she asked me what year it was – followed by the month – and even the day. I was doing pretty well with all the answers until the killer question came.

She asked me to spell the word WORLD backwards.

I tried D.R.L.O.W – but that wasn't right. So she decided I wasn't fit to be at large and gave me the option of either admitting myself for observation as a voluntary patient or being sectioned by her. I chose the voluntary option.

I was taken to a ward and had to hand in my belt and lighter. I was then shown my room, sparsely furnished with just a bed, chair and wardrobe. The widows didn't open. I still had my bag from the trip so I put some clothes in the wardrobe and put a few books on the shelves – most of them were R.D. Laing and similar psychology books. I also had some DVDs, including *One Flew Over the Cuckoo's Nest*.

I was having a cigarette in the outside smoking area, chatting to another patient who introduced himself as *Jesus of Stockport*. Jesus told me he had a haulage firm and could get me cheap trainers. He also told me he was an undercover officer working for the NHS to assess which patients were suitable for jobs in the outside world in his haulage firm. Even in my manic state I could clearly see through his delusions as he continuously begged patients for cigarettes. He watched me as I put my stub out in the ashtray and then walked over to retrieve it. There was still a full centimetre left, and that for him meant a treat with more puffs than usual.

Afterwards, a staff member called Bill – a short, rotund man with keys dangling from his belt – came into my room and said, "Come on, I'll show you round." The games room had a pool table with one cue and about six balls, a football table with three legs and a DVD player that didn't work. There was another lounge where patients sat watching *Jeremy Kyle* on television. John showed me the kitchen saying, "Make yourself a brew and join the others." A few residents were wearing dressing gowns. One girl had bandages on her wrists, while a lad opposite her had his head in his hands. Another chap was talking on a mobile phone to a girl who he was waving at through the widow in another ward on another floor. When we got talking he told me he had jumped off a motorway bridge after his girlfriend, who was the mother of his daughter, dumped him. Another chap sat on the settee playing his guitar. He appeared to be a gifted musician and after he finished playing he told me he took drugs in Thailand and had developed psychosis. He was really hyper, couldn't sit still and spoke very fast. Then the 6 o'clock medicine trolley was wheeled in and everyone got up from their seats and went to form a queue.

The word depression is wrong – totally wrong. It neither captures nor conveys the separation a person feels between them and the world. When I'm depressed, it feels like I'm possessed by something and there is a glass shield separating me from other human beings, which prevents me from reaching out and touching them. It is my experience that bipolar depression is double the strength of ordinary depression and completely paralyses the mind. It has nothing to do with feeling down, being a bit fed up, off colour, or any of the other hundreds of everyday descriptions associated with the word. You also have to wonder what triggers depression of this depth. I often think about the impact that 9/11 had on my consciousness and see how its horror was capable of activating trauma beyond my control. After all, the world changed that day. The sight of the planes going into the Twin Towers is etched in my memory. I've read since that a lot of mental illness was triggered by it. It had an impact on me because I thought the minute that it happened that it was an inside job, and still do. My reasoning was based on the stock market at the time, with the USA needing something to drag the markets out of a slump.

The media falsely portrays modern society as more at ease with discussing mental health than the previous generation, but this is not entirely true because bipolar episodes are not easy things to talk about. The stigma of having a mental health diagnosis travels with you and needs to be introduced to new partners, friends, employers, and so on. If you want to evaluate how much of a stigma is still attached to mental illness, ask any person who has been in a psychiatric hospital how many people came and visited them. The answer is usually none. It takes a few years to get back into life after a stay in hospital and receiving a diagnosis. Parts of what happened afterwards are still a blur because the medication made me sleep continuously. It is like having to clear up the mess of having your house flooded. In my case, once I established and gained insight and acceptance of my condition, I began the recovery process, starting with moving out of my brother's flat and into my own. I cut out alcohol and cannabis because both are detrimental to bipolar, with drinking in particular a bad combination. Once I had settled into my new home, I started rebuilding relationships with my children, which is an ongoing process.

I'm fully aware that I'm a manipulative old sod and control situations to my advantage with family, friends and even my landlord. Recently, I decided I needed a new carpet, so instead of paying the rent on time, I went and bought the carpet and had enough money left over to buy a shirt I wanted. Then there are times when I carry out pranks by pretending I'm going manic – or if I notice a shift in my mood, I'll make out it's worse than it is – either to test the will of somebody or because it's a good way of legitimising reckless behaviour, or excusing inappropriate temper outbursts, because people tolerate it if they think its connected to my bipolar. I do *ad hoc* work in the film industry and while I don't earn a fortune, it puts bread on my table. Bankruptcy took care of the debts. I no longer have a credit card. I don't have a pension either – nor savings. But I don't whinge, because I know that despite my misfortune,

I'm still a lot better off than other people. Now let me see – what would I change if I could re-live the last decade of my life? Well, the truth is, despite all the upheavals, debts, divorce, drama and hospitalisations, I wouldn't change a thing. It would be a waste of time me going over what I can't do anything about. I'm able to keep an eye on the present and hope for good things to happen in the future – but for me the past is done and dusted.

My top ten bipolar characteristics:

1. A professional mood watcher
2. Total avoidance of stressful situations
3. Constantly worrying
4. Irrationality
5. Low self-esteem
6. Ideas continuously flowing in my head
7. Maintaining the ballast of my ship
8. Self-efficacy and guilt
9. Obsessive tunnel vision
10. Learning from the mistakes of my past.

Ryan

Irene

I tried to open my eyes but they felt too heavy. I wanted to respond to the questions I was being asked, but couldn't find the words. The bed felt warm and cosy. I could see and sense people around the bed, yet my thoughts drifted off in another direction. I listened to someone screaming in the corridor, yet felt protected from harm. Sleep felt like the perfect option, my only desire, but they kept on talking.

"Irene, you've got to wake up and take your medication," said a voice.

I could feel my shoulders being shaken and a male voice saying, "I think one of the options is electric shock treatment." I didn't understand what he was saying. It was like he was speaking a foreign language. I opened my eyes and watched his mouth move. Unable to respond, my attention became transfixed on his turquoise tie with its light stripes, before closing my eyes again after a nurse had given me the tablets.

I could vividly see my brother Adrian standing by the front door of our parents' house, waving goodbye to me as I was been driven off in the back of my father's car. I could sense fear on my face and although I couldn't fathom out why I was feeling afraid or where I was being taken, Adrian's big smile and wave brought reassurance that everything would be okay. He smiled easily and often blushed at the same time, but it was these traits that endeared him to so many people. He is smiling in the photograph that my niece Doreen has of him on her mantelpiece, yet he looks younger now than in the photograph. It's as if he wants to take me back to when we were both in our twenties, to a time when we were both happy. I turn around to return his wave but instead hear the words, "It was a sin what he did – a sin". It was my mother's voice. She said this over and over again with the words 'a sin' ringing out so loudly, like they were spoken through a loudspeaker, making me want to cover my ears and scream "Stop!!!"

When I woke up, Doreen was sitting by my bedside. Her visits were the highlights of my days. I love her so much, but she doesn't understand my anguish. It irritated me when she would say, "You'll be better soon," like you'd say to a child who had fallen and grazed a knee. I heard her utter those words so many times and learned to just say, "I hope so," whenever they were spoken. Some days we would sit in the dayroom. I was only ever allowed out of my bedroom when Doreen came to visit. At all other times the door was locked, leaving me in a room that was little bigger than a tiny cage. The window in the room only opened a small amount, allowing little air to get inside. Every time I emerged from the room I felt freedom, in the same way I imagine prisoners must feel upon getting released from long periods of incarceration. We sat on the frayed settee in the dayroom, making idle conversation as we drank lukewarm tea from polystyrene cups, trying to ignore a fellow patient as her urine gushed down onto the floor. Nearby, an old man sitting in the corner mumbled to himself.

A nurse entered the room. "Irene, you need to return to your room to take your medication," she said.

"But I only took some an hour ago," I replied.

She ignored my protest and turned her back and left.

After I was discharged, I went to Doreen's home to recuperate after she kindly invited me, like she did on the other occasions when I had been in hospital. I decided it was the best thing to do until I was strong enough to return home by myself, although I never really felt at home there and often stayed in bed until three or four in the afternoon. I felt like I was under her family's feet and that I was only there because they pitied me. They often complained about me behind my back. I often overheard little remarks and one day I heard Doreen say to her friend that I was forever whinging about everything. She must have thought that I was asleep but I had got up to go to the bathroom. How dare she be so cruel? I glared at her and after her friend had left I said, "Is that what you really think of me?" But she didn't reply. Did she not realise that I was doing her a favour by staying with her? The house was full of germs. Her children were forever getting sick and passing on their illnesses to me. I woke up one morning with a terrible migraine. The day before that I had a terrible sore throat, no sooner than I had recovered from a cold passed on from Doreen's husband. How could anyone get well in that house?

I finally decided to return home. Doreen kept reminding me before I left to remember to take my medication. And of course she slipped in, "Now, you won't do anything silly," which we both understood to mean that I wouldn't commit suicide. That's the selfish side to Doreen. She wasn't thinking about me. She was thinking about herself and her family, thinking the stigma of another suicide in the family would be too unbearable to sustain. But little does Doreen know about the mental anguish that pushes someone to kill themselves. She's never endured the mental turmoil that Adrian went through, and Little Miss Perfect doesn't know what goes on in my head either. She says she understands me, but her patronising comments are far from convincing. Anyway, why should I care about what she thinks?

It couldn't have come at a better time. There was a permanent smile on my face as I read the wording on the invitation over and over again. My friend's son was getting married and this meant I needed to go shopping for new clothes. Yes, it was time to take my credit card shopping and coax some life back into it. I decided to go into the city, and made a list of the things I needed to buy. I had no time to waste and caught the mid-morning train. It was lunchtime when I arrived. I loved the buzz of the city, with everyone dashing about the place. I had awoken from my slumber like a tortoise on its first day out of hibernation.

I walked up and down every street, in and out of shops, yet failing to get the perfect outfit for the wedding, getting distracted in the process by an advertisement for Botox. A side-long glance in the mirror told me that my face definitely needed a little of this to get rid of the wrinkles and without a further thought I found myself sitting down having the treatment. Then I did more shopping. I managed to get a perfect pair of *Jimmy Choo* shoes. At first I had considered myself too old for such high heels, but the shop assistant assured me that I looked great in them. I agreed with her and bought a matching handbag as well. My hair was a total mess. I hurried back to the salon where I'd had the Botox and instantly booked myself in with a senior stylist for a complete makeover.

Then my mobile rang. It was Doreen, asking how I was.

"I'm terrific, my dear. I'm here in town, catching up on some retail therapy and treating myself to…"

But before I could continue she interrupted me. "Oh my God, are you sure you are alright?"

But I quickly replied, "I'm in the hairdressers, got to dash, bye bye, dear." It irritates me how she treats me like a baby and keeps checking up on me. I wish she would leave me alone and mind her own business once in a while. When I got out of the salon it was approaching closing time and I still hadn't managed to buy my outfit for the wedding. I felt my stomach churn with disappointment, but no sooner had this occurred that I passed a travel agent, advertising cheap flights to London with accommodation included. The travel agent arranged everything for me, although she was surprised that I wanted to leave for London later that evening.

"Have you got any ID on you?" she asked me.

"Yes, I have my driving licence," I replied.

I was on a mission and determined that nobody was going to stop me from going to London or having a good time. I bought a rucksack and put all my shopping bags in it before catching a taxi to the airport. It was brimming with crowds of people. I loved looking at the flight screen and seeing the list of destinations, making me realise that I wanted to travel more. Paris was easy to get to from London, and instantly the idea of going became stuck in my head.

I booked into a hotel close to Oxford Circus so that I could be near the shops. The next morning I left the hotel swiftly after breakfast and, judging by the number of shopping bags I acquired, did some serious retail therapy, including getting the ideal outfit for the wedding – a beautiful calf-length red chiffon dress that had sequins resembling small diamonds around the waist. Afterwards, I spotted a perfect pair of earrings that would match the dress, and decided to buy them.

"I'm sorry Madam, but your card has been declined," said the young man behind the counter.

"Are you kidding? Damn, what am I going to do?" I replied.

The streets were buzzing with activity, people dashing in all directions as I stepped out onto the pavement, digesting my bad news. I felt like a condemned woman, although I still managed to retain a feeling of surreal satisfaction that I had enjoyed such a good time all by myself. I had bought lovely clothes and accessories and felt I deserved all the treats I had lavished upon myself. After all, how often had the therapists told me that I should love myself more! I had laughed and joked with strangers and sampled the delights of London like a long-lost friend. I felt proud of my achievements, and to mark that great milestone I returned to the hotel and ordered room service. I smiled to myself, the condemned woman having her *last supper* before I mustered up the courage to ring Doreen and summon her help.

We flew home in silence. It was like her tongue had taken an unexpected rest but I discovered this was a short-lived reprieve until we arrived back home. During the car journey home, the first scolding was delivered, followed by a series of questions. When we arrived at her house, all my bags were opened and everything in them laid out. The interrogation went on for hours and included asking me how much everything had cost. There was only one way to quell the ranting and that was to go to bed – where I remained for three days. The beauty of silence was never more appreciated.

I still have the wedding to look forward to. It brightens up my waking moments and helps me to forget the dreadful Lithium and antidepressants that the cruel Doreen never forgets to place on my meal trays. On one of those occasions she announced, "I've cancelled your credit cards – you'll never be able to pull a stunt like that again." Then she threatened to stop me from going to the wedding, but the glare I gave her in return ensured she didn't try that a second time.

I intend going back to my own house shortly. The timing is good because her eldest son has his Leaving Certificate examination coming up, so she won't object. She will pretend to protest a little though, superficially, and will then relent after a few attempts. She will think she has beaten Auntie Irene. But neither Doreen nor anyone else will beat Auntie Irene. No indeed, because I will come up with another plan of action to strike back. Boxers get punched all the time during bouts and fall to the ground. Some get up and fight again whilst others just lay there, beaten. But I am like a boxer who hits the ground and then bounces back on his feet again and continues the fight. Surrender is not an option in his case and neither is it for me. The sooner that Doreen allows this to sink into her head, the better for all concerned.

Roger

It started after I came home from work one day after a particularly stressful shift as a civilian communications operator for the police. I had what I can only describe as a breakdown. I pushed all my family away from me. I became self-destructive, hell-bent on destroying my marriage and my relationships with everyone I knew. I started to drink heavily because it blocked out the feelings of despair I was having, although the alcohol actually made me feel far worse. I thought it was everybody else's fault, and not mine. On particularly bad days I started to self-harm, something I had never contemplated or done before in my life. I remember those dire days as being like a darkness closing in on me and I could do nothing to stop it. Although I tried to block everything out, it was still like sitting there with one's head inside a black cloud because nothing and no-one mattered anymore. I used to sit in the garden in front of a chimira, just staring into a fire holding a knife, which eventually I would use to cut myself. It was a way of relieving the intense feeling of pressure that had built up in my mind. If my wife tried to speak to me, I would just push her away, saying she didn't understand. When I was in these periods of darkness it felt very strange. I could sense she was there and talking to me, but she seemed very far away and when she spoke it didn't make any sense – it was almost as if I was underwater and she was trying to speak to me from the surface.

There were also times I had thoughts of ending it all; I felt worthless and a failure at everything I had done in life. It seemed pointless continuing, no matter what anyone said or did for me. This happened a number of times, and all the while it would be the same feelings of despair and worthlessness. I was planning to drive my car over a cliff but the one thing that kept me going was my daughter. I would see her face in my mind and would manage to stabilise myself enough to think about what it would do to her.

But how did my life descend into hell? Let me take you back to the beginning, to how it all started. I had a lovely childhood and what made it so special was that I had two loving, kind and remarkable parents as well as a twin brother and three sisters. We lived in a nice house and both my parents had good jobs. I went to good schools, played lots of rugby in scrum position, and had many friends. My parents, brother and sisters were a team and together we enjoyed great holidays every summer. We visited amazing places like Venice, Paris, Crete and Berlin as well as going camping annually to Scotland, where we used to camp near woods close to Loch Rannoch. Those were sometimes scary trips, but were also full of wonderment, especially having to cope with the darkness and silence of the woods at night, which encouraged my siblings to make scary noises, trying to convince me that wild animals were outside our tent trying to get in. Their games used to frighten me so much that I'd thought I'd have a heart attack, although in essence, everything was the epitome of happiness. But it was about that time, aged thirteen, that I made the discovery that would change my world and send me off on a difficult journey.

Retrospectively, the discovery changed my life instantly, although at the time I was not aware of the impact it was going to have on me. My outlook on life changed though, definitely changed from that day on.

My parents had an office at home and one day, whilst they were out, I went in looking for a pen or scissors, I can't remember which but what has remained clear is the shock I felt when rummaging through a drawer. I discovered a document which revealed that my brother and I were adopted. That was the moment that I realised that my life had been a façade. I wasn't really who I thought I was and neither was my twin brother. But if I wasn't who I thought I was, well then who was I? That I couldn't answer. There were no answers – only questions, but to ask them required courage. It took several years to summon up enough bravery to do so, but in the meantime I lived in limbo – afraid, lost and while surrounded by people who I knew and loved, I still felt a sense of abandonment from my real mother. But when I did eventually approach my adoptive parents, they were truthful, helpful and provided me with information that set about the search for my biological mother. Assisted by Social Services and the Adoption Contact Register, I gathered further information pertaining to my identity. But then I drew a blank. I was then in my late teens. A career in the navy beckoned. Hard work, lots of drink and a girl waiting for me at every port became my way of life for several years, but the feeling of wanting to know who my real mother was forever lurked in my mind, with heavy drinking never quite quenching the desire to find her – because the rationale was that if I found her, then I would find the real me. My career in the navy had its shelf-life, and when I returned to civvy street, I got married and had two children, a son and daughter. Loads of mundane jobs followed, but none of them quelled my curiosity to find my real mother and by the time I reached my thirties, the desire turned into an obsession.

My twin brother, on the other hand, felt very differently to me. From the very early days when my initial enquires into our adoption started, he made it abundantly clear that he had no interest in any of it. He was resolute that as far as he was concerned, our mother and father and sisters were the only family he had. I was somewhat surprised at his reaction, but respected the fact that he didn't share my thirst for knowledge and the need to know more about how we had started out in life.

To cut a very long story short, I eventually tracked down the woman who I wanted to meet more than any other person in the world. I found her through the modern advancement of internet searches, thanks to pointers given by the adoption agency and based on new information they had uncovered. She lived in New Zealand. My good luck didn't end there though because to my joy, I also discovered that my biological father was also alive and what's more, he was married to my real mother. Overnight, I went from not knowing who either of my biological parents were to having their email address and telephone number. I was beyond doubt that this wondrous unearthing could only mean that I was being led closer to finding the real me.

I arranged to call them, feeling like I had a date with destiny; finally, after forty years, I was going to speak to the person who gave me life. I thought my nerves were acting up before my phone call. I actually had to pluck up the courage to pick up the phone and dial the number. I had so many preconceived ideas about the situation that I found myself in, but in a split second they all paled into insignificance. There was a voice at the end of the phone saying, "Hello, my darling," a voice that although strange seemed familiar, but you just can't put your finger on it exactly. Although you actually know why, of course you do, how can you not? For me it was somewhat stranger, my birth mother had named me before putting me up for adoption and I was Roger, I had always known that but what I hadn't taken into consideration, of course, was that my birth parents had only ever known me as Graham and for forty years they had only ever referred to me as Graham.

Their names were Betty and James – my real mum and dad. I spoke to Betty on the telephone every week. James was very deaf and, although he came on the phone once, because of his disability we found it hard to communicate. There was seven months between finding them and meeting them. The anticipation of going to New Zealand and actually meeting them defied words. They held the missing link to the jigsaw puzzle. But this wasn't any ordinary puzzle. This was *my* puzzle. This was going to be my moment of finding completeness. I was quickly approaching my fortieth birthday, but in my heart I was still a little boy as I counted down the days when I would fly out with my wife and children to meet the couple responsible for giving me life. This is the email I sent them before I commenced the journey.

Dear Betty and James,

Overwhelmed and stunned at the moment, but in the best possible way in the world. You wonder what will happen and how you will react when your family make contact with the people who gave you the most precious gift of all, life. I have never doubted that you thought about me throughout our lives. It was the same for me, always wondering and hoping against all hope that this day would someday happen. I always understood the reasons why you had to give us up. Although I never knew the full details, I never felt any bitterness about the circumstances, just a quiet understanding as to possibly why. It could not be the easiest decision in the world to make, just the very fact you kept the birth tags and photograph tells me that. There are no burning questions that I need to ask and yet there are so many, forty years is a long time after all. I just have an overwhelming sense of relief I have found you and that you are there for me still. I guess you have a million and one things you want to ask me as well though. My biggest fear through all this was that if I found you, I would be intruding on someone else's lives. This has proved not to be the case.

The journey to New Zealand was long and the heat on arrival was stifling, even hotter was my eagerness to reach the moment that I had waited for all my life. Now I knew I was on its cusp. How did I feel? Excited, nervous, cautious, and happy. I experienced all of those but it was difficult to keep up with emotions as they darted about on the horizon by the minute, with me turning each one away because at their root was doubt. Some gut feeling was telling me that the trip wasn't going to be a success. That nagging gut instinct seemed to delight in torturing my mind with suspicion. When I first laid eyes on them, I felt nothing. There were no tears and little joy either, making it an anticlimax. It was just like meeting two strangers, albeit polite and welcoming, at least to begin with. The first evening in their home was congenial, but there was no depth to the conversation or opportunity to ask why they had given me and my brother up for adoption – and although there were promises given in emails to divulge this information during the visit, they weren't forthcoming that evening or any other – and to this day that question remains firmly unanswered. In addition to the less-than-exuberant reunion, there was a constant strain amongst us, which would eventually turn into a cold atmosphere in which none of us would feel comfortable in each other's company. But before that reached its peak we had to plough through much unpleasantness. Betty and James insisted on calling me Graham. I told them I didn't want this, as my adoptive parents named me Roger and this was the name I felt most comfortable being called. They ignored my request. When I told them things about my adoptive parents, they appeared disinterested or changed the conversation. Within hours of my arrival, they had arranged for the local newspaper to come to their home to tell the story of our reunion, but refused permission for my wife and children to be included in the photograph. That was the first instance of much exclusion for my wife and particularly my daughter, who was six at the time. They appeared to prefer my son, who was fifteen, and on several occasions remarked how spoilt they perceived my daughter to be, which wasn't the case. She missed home, had a stomach bug and I guess children are good at picking up bad atmospheres. Betty and James told me they wanted me to leave England and to go and live in New Zealand, where they would allow me to build a house on their land. While this might have been a kind proposal, and had it being given in different circumstances might have been one that I'd have considered, within days I appeared to be constantly arguing with them, especially over nasty remarks they kept making about my wife, saying she was fat and unattractive, and my daughter, whom they insisted was an attention-seeker. Thankfully, there was a lovely town and beach a couple of miles from where they lived, which acted as a bolthole for my wife, children and I to escape to each day. As the days went by we seemed to spend longer there, returning to their home after dark. But the stress of the situation became too much, prompting me to approach James and say that I felt it would be better if we went and stayed in a hotel for the remainder of our stay. He agreed. We packed up at once and when leaving, neither Betty nor James waved us goodbye. After I returned home, my anger surged to great heights. The whole trip appeared to have been a waste of time. I felt I was no closer to the truth than before and also thought that I was further away from finding my real self than at any other time in my life. In haste and anger, I sent Betty and James an email expressing my disquiet.

Dear Betty and James,
Make of this what you will, just be mindful of the fact
that I did all the running in this voyage of discovery.
I was the one who phoned every week to talk to you
and made the plans to come out and see you and I did
it all with genuine love and absolutely honesty. It was
you who decided that certain members of my family
were 'distractions' and stopped us talking. Nothing
could be further from the truth. Those members of
the family were made to feel uncomfortable and
unwanted from more or less day one and trust me,
I know what you truly think of 'the females' and I
would not and could not allow them to feel that way
so far away from home. You never appreciated that
my daughter was only six, a long way from home,
from her friends, family and home comforts that
make a child comfortable in their environment. You
excluded her and yet you had the audacity to heap
loads of love and attention on her brother whilst she
was in the same room. That was nothing short of
outrageous; you treated my family whilst we were
in your care abysmally.

You see adoption stories on television and marvel, even cry
at the happy outcome when sons and daughters are reunited
with their parents. Forgiveness and understanding are
readily available and so too seem to be the answers behind
each adoption. Well not for me, you will never see my story
on television because the ending is far too miserable to put in
a programme. The years passed quickly after my disastrous

trip to New Zealand and, in one sense, I put the whole thing to one side because I had begun to think that my identity was a mess, that I would never discover who I really was and basically had given up on life. I became increasingly angry about my childhood and found myself constantly thinking about how and why I had so many regrets about events in my life. I had begun to question everything about my existence; my relationship with my adopted family was by then at an all-time low. I had made up my mind that I didn't want to have anything to do with them ever again because they never asked me about what happened in New Zealand after I returned. Every time I spoke to them or met up with them, we argued, I accused them of letting me down because I knew my relationship with them would never be the same as it used to be and I didn't care. I was in self-destruct mode and drank lots and lots of whiskey.

I was also angry that I hadn't listened to the adoption agency who had advised me to take things slowly after I found out the identity and location of my real parents. I was told it was unwise to meet them at their home in the first instance and that it would be best to meet on neutral territory, just by myself, rather than taking along my wife and children. But I thought I knew best. The telephone calls and emails had lured me into a false sense of security. Besides, I was headstrong and have in life tended to do things in haste, never quite thinking about the consequences until afterwards, when it is usually too late. But I started to wonder if I could undo some of this wrong. What if I tried again? I contemplated contacting them a second time and asking them if we could start afresh. I even thought about picking up the telephone and apologising. In my mind, I began to plan another visit to rectify some of the harm, make amends, find answers – and ultimately acquire inner peace in my quest to discover the true me. But around the time I was ready to act, I received an email from a legal firm informing me of their deaths, which occurred within six months of each other. This was the worst possible thing that could have happened and made me sink into the worst depression of my life. I became paralysed with fear and regret. I appeared to have lost everything and there was nobody in my family to whom I could reach out for support. I had destroyed all my relationships and were it not for the love and iron will of my wife who stood by me, I would have destroyed her and my children as well.

After eventually being diagnosed with bipolar, I was put on Diazepam and Citalopram, which helped to blank out my thoughts. I hated taking medication at first, but now I'm used to it. I have now been discharged by the crisis team and am currently about to undergo Cognitive Behavioural Therapy. I am happier than I have been, but I still have bad days, although apparently this is to be expected. I am told that with therapy things should become easier. I am hopeful the therapy will put my life into perspective and will help untangle the chaos in my mind, because as in the words of the rapper Eminem's 1990s hit record: ....*cause I'm Slim Shady, yes I'm the real Shady, all you other Slim Shadys are just imitating, so won't the real Slim Shady please stand up, please stand up, please stand up?*.......... Who is the real me? The real me is Roger – not Graham. It took me a while to realise this, and for a while I deliberated about who I thought I might be. But I grew up Roger, got married, had children and I am still that person. I just had a different name after I was born and yes, life would have been very different if I had remained Graham and lived his life. My life has consisted of a few blips and a bit of a bumpy ride at times but no worse than anyone else who hasn't been adopted. As with everybody, life is not always perfect, but I am happier these days with who I am and what I have become – and where my life has taken me. I think I am growing at peace with myself and appreciate that what I discovered about my identity was like a jigsaw that just needed putting together. The jigsaw is coming along nicely now, and pieces are fitting together. Bipolar is just a piece of this jigsaw, like all the other pieces. My job now is just to put it in its right place and move forward with my life.

What bipolar means to me:

1. Imposed exile
2. A mirror of other people's discontent
3. Being a visionary
4. Close to nature
5. So sensitive that I become skinless
6. Carelessness (I don't have care in the world when manic)
7. Surprising
8. We are all a mixture of darkness and light
9. Interesting
10. Unfair and never ending

Annette

Natasha

I attempted suicide three times – twice by overdosing and once when I slit my wrists, which left a big scar on one of them. I constantly have to make excuses when inquisitive people ask me what caused it. Although I've had thoughts of killing myself when depressed, these have never been acted upon. Surprisingly, all of my suicide attempts occurred when I was in a manic state.

I was new to London when I first tried to kill myself. It was after I left my hometown in County Wexford and went to work in London that I first started the whole nightclub partying scene that involved taking cocaine most nights, often leaving me confused, dazed and full of torment.

Diary extract – Suicide Attempt One:
It wasn't like any of my other drunken nights. From the outset this was different. My boyfriend and I got wine and were like knackers drinking down some alleyway. The alleyway was actually really pretty though. It looked like it was straight out of the 1800s. I really liked just being there with him, talking. It was so nice as we were the only people there and not one person walked past us. On the other side of the road, a mouse ran out from somewhere and ran along the side of a building and into a tiny hole. We were drinking from a wine bottle. He said, "I love you." It was so great to hear. I was pretty drunk at

this stage and I don't remember if I told him I felt the same way or not.

Later that night, a friend called me to say her grandmother had died. I decided that I should go around to her house and comfort her. When I arrived she was doing cocaine, and I had some too. I drank some wine as well, and my mind was getting really hazy by now. She got out a box full of Xanax and offered me some. I took a few, I don't know how many or why. I asked her if I could keep the rest and she said yes. I then started to feel sick. I got a taxi to my boyfriend's house, but in the back of the cab I continued on taking the pills. I didn't want to 'be' alive anymore. I don't know what triggered this thought, but I felt my time was up and genuinely believed this was the right thing to do. When I got to my boyfriend's place he paid for the taxi. I then went into his flat and fell to the ground and my next memory was waking up in hospital.

I was fed a cocktail of drugs, resulting in the days that followed being spent either crying or sleeping, but eventually I bullshitted my way out of hospital. I'm good at bullshit, and convinced the medical team that I only took cocaine because I was drunk, which in turn lead to me taking the Xanax – and promised them that I'd never do it again. It worked, and soon afterwards I was discharged with a prescription for antidepressants. When I told my parents that I had been in hospital they pleaded with me to return home and offered to send me money.

I remember my flight home on Aer Lingus because I cried the whole way home. I was at rock bottom and felt I had failed in life. It was about three or four days before my family said I had started to return to normal. Whatever normal was for me. My parents arranged for me to see a clinical psychologist. She spoke with me for over an hour but I just cried and cried before she suggested that I went to the psychiatric hospital for treatment, which I refused to do. I know I put my family through hell. My mother was in pieces and cried whenever she saw me. My brother understood my torment and was extremely supportive – and so was my dad, who offered to pay for private care to get me better again.

My moods were up and down and, although I tried to mask them in front of my family, the pressure inside me kept building up – so I decided to move to the city to start a new job. My situation didn't improve, and although I wasn't taking drugs any longer, I was drinking excessively. I stopped taking the antidepressants, which was a big mistake because a manic episode followed, and once again I attempted suicide and ended up being sectioned in hospital. My life felt absolute shit. But once again I lied my way out of the situation. It wasn't difficult. I told the doctors what they wanted to hear and soon afterwards I was discharged again with another prescription for antidepressants and an antipsychotic. Despite this, my drinking continued.

Diary extract – Suicide Attempt Two:
Now it's Saturday night. There is a party in a friend's
house for another friend's birthday. At the party I
was drinking from the punch bowl like it was water

because I was very thirsty. I felt I had to finish what I started. I wasn't meant to be here. I just remember feeling so intense. Not frightened though. This was right for me. I called home, and I spoke with my parents and brother. Afterwards, I decided I needed to go and end my life. So I snuck out of the party, turned my phones off and went into the night. Hoping to disappear forever, I overdosed again on Xanax. I popped my pills out of their packets, all of them – I think a month's supply, or more even. And I took them all. I then went and lay on my bed and held a teddy bear that I had had since I was a small girl. Not a lot went through my mind. I just waited. I was at peace. It was short-lived. My roommate found the empty pill packets and asked me what I had done. I insisted that they were just empty packets but she called an ambulance anyway. Soon, it came and the paramedics asked me what I had taken. I refused to go with them; however they told me if I didn't cooperate that they'd call the police, who'd make me go. When I got to hospital I was given activated charcoal and vomited up the pills.

I don't know what caused my bipolar. I had a happy childhood – nice parents who have always been supportive and likewise a brother who is good to me. I never had any trauma that could be linked to me feeling the way I do. Every psychologist I've seen has asked me the same patronising questions about my upbringing and schooling. They constantly sniff away at my background, looking for something upon which to pin my moods. I tell them a little tale about withdrawing from life when I was in my fifth year at school. It's a true one but I doubt if it has any great relevance to me becoming bipolar later on in late teens. I was always academically gifted but during the years between my junior and leaving certificate, I became depressed. I resented the way I was always the top student in my class but never really got the credit for it. Looking back, I was looking for validation at the time. I would be the happiest person ever one week, and the next I'd be grumpy and depressed – but is there a teenager that doesn't experience those type of moods?

The psychiatrist I saw when I got back from London firmly believed that medication was the answer to treat what she called my 'chemical imbalance'. That was the first time I had heard this term, and there was something in her tone of voice that made me think there was nothing other than medication that would help me. A glance around the room reinforced this belief when I noticed brand names of drugs everywhere in the room – on the clock, on her pen and even her mouse-pad had the name of a drug embossed on it. But the antidepressants she prescribed made my mind blurry and slowed me down completely, making my personality unpredictable. My mood swings intensified, making several friends abandon me after I made nasty comments about the way they looked, their partners, children and so on. If I woke up and fancied not going to work that day I never had the slightest hesitation about calling in sick.

Diary extract – Suicide Attempt Three:
I was on a range of pills for a few months. None really agreed with me and again after another great

night out, feeling on top of the world (and with a bit of Dutch courage) I decided that my time was up. I took a taxi home from town and I had the taxi driver stop at an ATM where I took my cash limit out and gave all the money to him. He was from Nigeria and told me a sad story about how he struggled to pay bills and support his wife and family. I knew I was going to die that night, so I gave him my money. I went into my kitchen when I got home and opened a bottle of wine. Again I believed that this was the best thing for me to do. I didn't actually think of my family or anyone else. I didn't really think of anything, just killing myself. I don't believe in God or anything so I believed that I was just going to be gone. And I was okay with that. I took a knife and started to cut my wrists. I felt no pain, but then my mother walked in and gasped in horror when she saw all the blood.

Shortly afterwards, my parents paid for me to see a private psychiatrist, costing them several hundred euros per hourly session. I initially saw him every week for a few months. I got on well with him. He told me that medication was a lazy remedy but that I might not have to take the pills forever – rather, firstly I'd need to be able to be talk more honestly about my feelings. He too believed, like my previous psychiatrist, that it was a chemical imbalance in my brain that had caused my bipolar and suicidal actions, and I guess he too made me accept this as the reason. The antidepressants, mood stabiliser and sleeping tablets continued to be prescribed, making me wish and hold on to the hope – back then as much as now – that the day will come when my brain mends itself of the imbalance and I no longer have to rely on these dreadful drugs.

I don't really like to use the word 'manic' and never use this word to describe myself to friends, because I don't feel comfortable using it. I prefer to just say 'up'. Manic to me seems to suggest something a bit drastic – although I know my actions when I'm *up* are drastic. Each time I am *up*, I'm in a really great place and everything is fantastic, I'm excited, happy, on a really good 'buzz', not from drugs or anything, just from my own *up*. The problem for me though is when I am in an *up* phase I can never imagine what it is like to be depressed, and vice versa. I can only compare it to finishing an enjoyable meal and finding it difficult to imagine what it is like to be hungry. The coin of my life gets continuously flipped – but I have learned over the years to take care of myself and to step back if a particular set of events begin to trouble me in some way.

My friends find it difficult to understand me and often accuse me of narcissistic tendencies as they claim, either rightly or wrongly, that I am consumed by my emotions – and sometimes give little in the way of attention to them. I am fun though, that is acknowledged. I am adventurous too. Last year I challenged a few of my friends to take a week off work and coaxed them into joining me on a *grande* tour of Ireland. We stayed in lovely hotels and guesthouses, climbed mountains and swam in rivers and lakes. We laughed, chatted to strangers wherever we went, ate and drank and smoked and sang. It was blissful, and we ended up seeing all thirty-two counties by the end of the week.

During my *ups* I have been overly promiscuous, shopped excessively, led myself into dangerous situations, been incredibly outgoing, drunk excessively, pushed things to the limits. But as it stands, I'm glad I've been through all of that. I've done things that I guess a *normal* person wouldn't do and say. I've gained an understanding into the world of mental problems which, in Ireland, people just refer to as 'troubles with their nerves'. Although it's regrettable how I've sometimes hurt people along the way, particularly my mother, I'm still here – and right now I want to be 'still here' for quite some time. I believe I am a much stronger person – stronger than a lot of people I know, making me feel glad that I failed three times to successfully kill myself.

Paul

I practiced holding the knife to my throat because I wanted to get used to the feel of its blade. Just one almightily forceful slice across the jugular vein would have meant enough bleeding to end my misery. But I'm a coward and deep down always knew I hadn't enough courage to go through with it. Besides, Hinduism believes if you commit suicide, you come back as a ghost. I have my own theory on suicide – if you rent a property, it becomes your liability if you deliberately set fire to it. God rents out your body to you. You don't own it – so if you destroy it, you pay a price in the afterlife.

I screamed constantly from birth up until the age of three every time I came into contact with cigarette smoke – which was, so I'm told, because my parents both smoked. Nevertheless, my mother brought me up well and all my friends at primary school referred to me as the *posh* kid. The fact that I came from a council estate escaped their attention. I was a bright child, with an advanced vocabulary for my years. I often got teased by my classmates: "Have you swallowed a dictionary?" But later on, my contemporaries at grammar school were less kind and referred to me as the *poor* kid. They were right. There was little money in our house. My father separated from my mother when I was seven. He said he'd come back, but as time went by it became clear he had reneged on his promise. But that didn't stop me hoping that one day he'd reappear. I left school when I was seventeen because the pressure of studying for A-levels became too much. By that stage, I had begun to smoke pot and drink cheap lager. They became a release for years of unexpressed anger. I have come to the conclusion over the years that everyone with bipolar is screwed up in some way or another. I blame my parents, particularly my mother, for messing up my life. When I was told my father had died, the news came with a double bomb-shell; my older sister told me that he had sent me cards, letters and presents every year for my birthday and Christmas, but instead of my mother telling me they were from him, she said they were from someone else.

My mother worked hard to provide for my sister and passed on to me her staunch socialist views. Although she failed to keep me away from religion, despite espousing disdain at religion and claiming it was rubbish. Instead of agreeing with her views, I made a point of reading the Bible and quoting passages to annoy her. I drifted from job to job in my late teens to early twenties; I became transfixed by politics and social justice and despised Margaret Thatcher's government and for a while couldn't speak about anything else. I remember going to the Poll Tax demonstrations in London in the late eighties and witnessing the sickening brutality of the police as they beat up a man for challenging them during the march. Around that time I moved out of home and started living in squats. The jobs I held were all low paid – bar work, cleaning jobs and working in factories. By the time I reached my twenty-second birthday I counted the number of jobs I'd had and laughed when the number matched my age.

One day, I was walking down Oxford Street when a Hare Krishna monk gave me a copy of the *Bhagavad-Gita*. This aroused my interest, prompting me to read ferociously on Hinduism. I accepted an invitation to the Hare Krishna temple in Soho and became so engrossed in its teaching and philosophy that I joined within six months. A new life started making me feel I was on the road to happiness and, to begin with, I was genuinely contented. I stopped smoking and drinking. I became a vegetarian and had to forego sex. I loved the routine and devotion of being part of a religious movement, and felt absorbed by the discipline of having to get up every morning at 4am to chant and sing for four hours before breakfast. But within a year, I started to become restless. The regime turned out to be impersonal. Celibacy was one thing, but not being allowed to masturbate caused frustration. However, the decision to leave was taken out of my hands. I suddenly stopped sleeping and after a week the insomnia became manic. Hare Krishna spoke about compassion and forgiveness, but another aspect to the movement is the business side. There is no room in it for sick people. Their philosophy was simple: 'no lazies and no crazies' – having endured enough of both during the sixties with acid-prone hippies. You were there to carry out a job – you were given a role – and once you became unable to fulfil that obligation, you ceased to be of use to them.

Life in psychiatric care has improved over the years, but back in the mid-nineties, hospitals were full of old-fashioned psychiatrists and male nurses who preferred to sit and read their newspapers than talk to patients. I was given an old, style atypical antipsychotic – Chlorpromazine – that made every muscle so stiff I walked like an old man ridden with arthritis. It slowed me down and it slowed the time down. After discharge, the Hare Krishnas refused to let me live in my previous accommodation at the temple, but instead directed me to share a caravan with another disciple. We were dispatched to France to spread the words of Krishna. It felt good living a carefree bohemian lifestyle and enabled me to learn fluent French. All was going well until I had another breakdown, rendering me surplus to requirements once again, so I was promptly dispatched back to England to seek treatment. I was hospitalised again for the standard twenty-eight days. This time I was given Olanzapine, which wasn't therapeutic in the least. It suppressed the functioning of the brain, made me lethargic and so hungry that I used to eat a loaf of bread in between meals. Is it any wonder people become fat and diabetic? But taking oral medication was better than being forcibly injected, which was comparable to being drugged to comatose level. That happened a few times when I refused medication. The staff, usually three or four burly nurses, would restrain me by throwing me to the ground and push down on pressure points on my arms to ward off my defence. It was done with such force that I was often left with bruising to my shoulders as well as to my arms. On one of those occasions I slept for days afterwards, making my blood pressure drop so dangerously low that I nearly ended up being transferred to a general hospital. The strange thing is that I firmly believe I would have got better without medication during those hospitalisations.

The routine of rest, regular meals and being with people who listen is often more than enough to resume stability in a manic person.

This pattern continued every year for twelve consecutive years, each year I would reliably turn up to hospital for my annual *vacation*. And then the cycle broke, not because there was a change in my circumstances, rather the system was less keen to hospitalise people, preferring to treat them at home instead. The irony was that once I was discharged I would instantly become medication-free – until the next incarceration. The one exception was when I agreed to take Mellaril, but that came to an abrupt halt after it was taken off the market for reportedly causing heart disease.

The only sensible words I've ever heard a psychiatrist speak were when he said to me: "Listen – 80% of this behaviour is simply you, it is your character – the other 20% is your bipolar and that is what I am treating with medication."

When the weather is hot in summertime, I lay on my bed looking out at the rays. The background sound of the radio helps fill the void. I search for answers to questions that cannot be answered: 'Why am I alive?' 'Why do I have to cope with this?' 'Who cares?' Apathy is ever-present, joined by its friend hopelessness. The high aspirations and ideals of my youth vanished, replaced by lonesome regrets. If I hadn't being so hot-headed and left school early, Oxford would have beckoned after having passing its entrance exam. Life could have been so different, but alas the grandeur of what eluded me was replaced with a lifestyle financed by benefits, a council property with unsavoury neighbours, a decade and a half of unemployment, no friends – unless I count the druggies and dregs who try to befriend me, and no one to love me because I'm unable to reciprocate. Basically, I am destitute in the broadest sense of the world – and nobody gives a damn. There are lucid moments during these catatonic emotional states, when a trip to the lavatory or kitchen helps to shake me out of my trance, but not without moments of indecision. Sometimes I go into the kitchen and open the cupboard with dread, trying to decide what to eat, and often, when unable to choose something, I don't bother, and return upstairs to bed. On good days, I stay up and watch television or play computer games. Other times I read, and if the book is interesting, I won't put it down until it's finished. My flat will be a complete mess but I won't care because I'm the only one who sees the stinking dishes in the sink – or tolerates the body odour of not having bathed or changed my clothes in months. The over-riding feeling that life is going to be shit anyway is why I don't care about myself. This hopelessness has at its core the belief that I am worthless, because optimism is afraid to come near me, preferring to detour instead in case it gets caught in the spider's web of my life. This is not living – it is an existence. And if it weren't for the fact that the Government pays my rent and that I receive Disability Living Allowance, death would be the only attractive option.

I am a fully confirmed recluse these days. I've remained a vegetarian, but rely mainly on tinned food because of infrequent trips to the supermarket. I still crave female company, but I haven't had a girlfriend in two years, around the time I last became manic. However, the truth is I find the intensity of sharing my life – my space – and my time too overbearing. Mania makes me say harsh, unpleasant things because my arrogance takes over, making me believe I'm invincible. That's why my girlfriend left me. It's not just the insults that cause havoc, because during mania I jump from topic to topic and switch to subjects completely irrelevant to the conversation. If I see a cloud in the sky that I think is at the wrong angle, I interpret this as a signal of some global plot. It's hardly surprising that nobody has enough stamina to tolerate such nonsense. So, two years ago, I retreated to home and battened down the hatches. I began taking a self-prescribed compilation of remedies including St. John's Wort and Ginseng, which help keep depression at bay. I also take Valerian, which is a herbal medicine with anti-anxiety properties – and Ayurvedic and Smriti Sagar which are alternative medicines believed to cure insanity and insomnia. This way I avoid upsetting people, I avoid embarrassment but most advantageous of all is that I have nobody telling me how to live or not live my life. That's the plus side of things. The part that isn't so good is that I have become totally risk averse, fearing failure so vehemently that I cannot do anything that risks me getting stressed, which invariably leads to long bouts of depression. In other words, my life is in limbo and for some reason, I receive fulfilment in knowing that while things can't get better this way, it's also unlikely they'll get any worse.

My bipolar is:

1. Maddening
2. Unquiet
3. A lens through which to view the world differently
4. Gladdening
5. As much a part of me as my blue eyes
6. Overwhelming at times
7. A word – not a sentence
8. Inspiring
9. Being different
10. Incessant.

Karl

Geraldine

*Psychiatrists all seem to go by the book on medication,
which makes me wonder why they take so long to
study the brain and then constantly give out the same
tablets. With all the research in the medical field, it
is amazing that mental health is not progressing,
which is a sad state for us sufferers.*

I was born in a rural part of Ireland, where my parents
ran a small business. I was the youngest of seven children
but despite a busy household, we had lots of fun as kids
and every one of us helped out in our own different way
to assist our parents. Education was deemed important –
we attended boarding school and most, including myself,
attended university. My family placed a huge importance
on money and achieving success in life. I left college in the
early eighties with an average result. The country was in
deep recession, with many economic challenges at the time,
and I returned home to live with my parents, where some
of my older siblings were also still residing. This made it a
stressful house, not least because it was a relatively small
bungalow. Bickering, rivalry and backstabbing were accepted
as normal behaviour, and became woven into our family
environment. My family had experienced a major fire a year
and a half earlier, in which much of my father's warehouse
was destroyed. My father was an extremely hard worker and
blamed himself for being negligent and causing the disaster.

This rubbed off on all the family, but especially those based at home who bore the brunt of his guilt and regret, resulting in him becoming harder to live with. I really wanted to move out, which I thought would help but there were absolutely no suitable jobs for graduates and the current support system for unemployed people was not in place in those days. The Sunday papers were full of stories from local fathers who were working in America, or elsewhere, trying to support their families back home. All the young people from my area left to go abroad and indeed many families emigrated too. Things were really desperate.

Time passed and I plodded along but became very depressed about my situation. The mood around me was very much doom and gloom, as well as the familial conflict. My parents didn't seem to be aware of my plight, or maybe they just hoped it would go away. This initially manifested as low mood – all the colour had gone from my life. I had a general feeling of despair and of being trapped and felt cut off from my friends. I felt no hope for the future, wishing my life away. I wasn't living and had no zest or enthusiasm for anything, as well as being mostly tearful. I easily entered into verbal conflict with siblings because of my low self-worth. Then I started to isolate myself even more and spent a lot of time in my bedroom. I became further detached from family members and friends, daydreaming in my bedroom, not living in the present, and not wanting to dress up or buy new clothes or go outdoors. I spent my days in bed or just walked around the house in my nightwear and ate very little.

I felt no-one cared about me and that I was doomed, which meant only bad things would happen to me. This, combined with a frightened and agitated state, led to me having bad dreams. I somehow knew that I was experiencing mental health issues, but found it difficult to put into words how I felt. I had a terrible pain in my head and I felt that it was going to shatter and burst. I was fearful about what was happening to me and terrified of having to be admitted to a mental hospital. I felt the whole of my life flashing though my mind and only saw the negative elements of my existence. I felt doomed and couldn't ever see myself conducting a 'normal' life again. I was terrified and felt I was falling apart mentally. I couldn't sleep and kept recounting all the terrible things that had ever happened to me. Negativity was constantly at the forefront of my mind. I never harmed myself and neither was I considered a danger to others, although my parents became extremely worried and thought I was having a nervous breakdown. I was taken to a psychiatrist the next day and she prescribed some mediation, which my mother gave me every day. The situation turned from bad to worse and I became acutely psychotic. My parents were extremely worried and shut me away in my room, terrified that anyone would find out that their daughter was 'mad'.

I was hospitalised for a few months, the first of many admissions, but I survived that and many more depressive episodes over the years. While my bipolar started with episodes of depression, it later progressed to manic episodes. My mania always presents itself with an abundance of energy. I never get tired, but those around me usually become fatigued by my behaviour. I can stay up half the night writing letters of complaint to various organisations about their services. Even when I'm well – as I am now – I love fighting for justice in the world. I'm not talking about something on a global scale – rather local community causes. But during the throes of mania, I am confrontational and rude. As well as writing letters, I constantly use the phone.

I'll never forget the time, during a manic episode, that I turned against my local parish priest because I disapproved of his fundraising methods for a new church roof – much to the horror of some of my fellow parishioners. One Sunday after Mass, he was standing at the church door as people were leaving,, shaking hands and patting babies on their heads. He looked at me as I drew nearer. "Geraldine, how are you?'" he asked and extended his hand out to shake mine. I looked to one side, raised my hand in a defensive stance and said, "Please don't speak to me," before walking straight past him.

I was so annoyed at what I considered his lacklustre approach. I felt the appeal needed more energy, commitment and leadership and what I saw in him was a laid-back, almost lethargic way of going about things. The blood in my body was pumping at double its usual speed when I discovered the few low-level events in the planning, which if left that way would have taken until doomsday to get enough funds to replace the roof. I decided it needed a more authoritative approach, so I contacted the local newspapers and radio station. I did interviews and talked about the history of the church and the importance and respect that the people it served held for it. I also wrote letters to newspapers overseas, as well as making hundreds of phone calls to local councillors and representatives, urging their financial support through applications for grants and various bursaries. It was very hard work but it paid off because within two years the parish

Geraldine

council had secured sufficient funds to call in the builders. By that time I was on speaking terms with the priest again.

When I'm manic I am indifferent to what people think of me. But whether or not my energy and motivation is driven by mania, I usually get a mixed reaction to my vocal personality. Some agree with me and tell me I'm doing the right thing. Others have expressed dismay because they are normally accustomed to pacifism in their lives and therefore I often get remarks from women of my own age who say to me, "I could never say the things you say," or "I would never do that in a million years." But I have no problem standing up for the things I believe in and will readily speak out to those who expect silent subservience because they think they'll get away with it.

Patients in psychiatric hospitals have a tremendous amount of spare time on their hands. The days are long, motivation is low, and freedom feels like a rich man's dream. Your independence, your power, your dignity, your self-respect is taken away and replaced with a strict regime, authority, detachment, shame and endless medication. During these long disempowered periods of time, you notice how patients interact with each other and what type of relationship the staff have with their patients. You observe the words they use, their tone of voice, their facial expressions and the warmth that a tactile hand brings when words are not needed or desired. I saw the way they treated Tom. I listened to what they said to him. I felt their cruelty. I loathed the powerlessness of not being able to help. The fear of the whistle-blower's punishment (which would undoubtedly have been an injection and extra medication).

The next step up from being in a straightjacket is an induced coma. The thought of a comatised existence brings the sort of fear that I can only imagine is felt by prisoners on death row.

Tom presented as a shy, well-groomed and unassuming man, a bachelor, of farming background who was in his early seventies. I saw him being hustled into the ward by two staff members with the distinctive sound of the key being clunked in the ward door as it locked. Tom seemed astonished to find himself in this situation. I could tell he was manic by the way he paced up and down the corridor, restless, scared and confused. Every time the door opened Tom rushed towards it trying to escape, but was grabbed by his arms and jostled back into the ward by male staff. He enquired of staff when he would be allowed out, saying that he had business to attend to. Their vocabulary was devoid of kind and reassuring words, they wore the look of ignorance on their faces with pride, but one of them eventually replied, "Will you wait a while? What's your hurry? You've just landed, haven't you?'

The hours turned into days. Tom was put on a lot of medication. He was still worried about his dog and his farm, his belongings and when he would be released. But his fears were not comforted with kindness, only nastiness. One of the male nurses used to whistle and call out "Prince!" or make clicking noises after he discovered the name of Tom's sheep dog, before bursting into laughter when he saw how disorientated Tom became when he did this. It was horrible to witness, and the thought of them thinking we were oblivious to their cruelty was equally hard to tolerate. Tom was often confined to his locked single room, an extremely small space with a cement-like painted floor, for long periods of time, and each time he emerged from his room he looked physically worse. The window in the room was sealed shut, with no fresh air supply. I know this since I was imprisoned in an identical room next to it. The radiators in the bedrooms were never switched off, even in summertime, making it stiflingly hot all the time. The doors usually remained locked. When Tom would emerge from the tiny room for short periods he was placed in a special chair and restrained with a belt. His health continuously deteriorated and he was placed on a nebuliser, a dirty machine that had been circulating around the ward and had been previously used by others and left on a window ledge in the day room. After a short few weeks, Tom became incontinent. One night, I peered through his door's tiny window and saw him lying there on the rough floor clad only in a nappy. A couple of days later he died.

Dinosaurs may be extinct, but their DNA lives on in the staff in mental hospitals. They are easily the most inquisitive and conniving group of people imaginable, who constantly invaded my privacy by wanting to know details about the house which they knew I owned – as well as the rest of my assets, bank account details and the names of who I would bequest my estate to in the event of my death. I strictly refused to disclose this personal information, because I knew the reasoning behind their questions. All you have to do is look at the historical nature of these hospitals to realise that their wealth was built up as a result of them being beneficiaries from patients they cajoled into giving them money. They like dependency. Mental hospitals have always meant big business and large-scale employment. My friends and I named the hospital where we were incarcerated, 'The Club', because generations of families worked there – couples, sons and daughters, brothers and sisters, in-laws of every description, neighbours and friends. Constant gossip, constant whispering and sharing of information existed among its 'members'. It had massive grounds and a big playing pitch where the children of the staff played. It ran itself entirely on the motto 'it's not what you know, but who you know', and felt threatened if strangers from outside the area joined its ranks.

My greatest fear is of having to ever go back to that awful place again, knowing that, if that happened, I would be given further medication and I know how detrimental that would be to my health. The last time they put me on Risperidone, which caused me to have hallucinations, to which they later admitted in a review meeting that I was allergic. During manic phases, which required me to be hospitalised, I used to ask for the police to accompany me to hospital because I wanted them to come inside and see how awful the place was, with the hope they'd report it to the relevant authorities and have the place shut down. I know how naïve that sounds but over the years I have come to realise that psychiatrists are above the law and can do whatever they like. I will also never forget the cavalier response I got from one staff member when I told him I was unhappy with my medication and the way he was treating me – and how I intended to report him to the HSE. I got a cold stare before he said, "You can report me to whomever you like, bring it on."

My GP though has great expertise in the area of mental health and has a practical approach, which is sadly lacking in other services. Rather than the customary textbook psychiatric question, "How is your mood?" we discuss practical issues around exercise and fitness plans, problems with weight and medication, how I'm managing at home, plans for holidays and how I'm getting along with my neighbours. He says that, in his opinion, exercise is one of the best methods for keeping well in mind and body. He promotes walking and swimming, but mostly walking because it is free to all. He is conscious that a lot of people who suffer mental health problems are on low incomes and gives advice on healthy eating. I have often been given advice during a visit for a meal that evening. An example of his recommendation would be: "Get a little piece of steak or a homemade burger off the meat counter in your local supermarket, select some fresh vegetables or salad and together with some oven chips you will have a decent, inexpensive meal in twenty minutes."

Over the years, remissions have come and gone but during one of the calm interludes I met my husband, who was a lovely, kind and supportive man. But after I gave birth to our son, our marriage fell apart when I went to pieces with the greatest bout of depression I had ever experienced in my life. I constantly felt I was in the middle of a thick fog, alone, cold and lost. The darkness of night further hindered the visibility, leaving me in a position where I could no longer imagine a glimmer of light ever appearing in my life again. Months passed and I still felt the same way. It broke me down, left me withered like a vase of flowers left without water in the sunshine. But there was no sunshine in my life or my marriage and eventually my husband and I decided to separate. There were no arguments or bitterness between us – just sadness that it had to end but with a silent understanding that it was in both our interests to go our different ways.

It was difficult to get back on my feet after the break-up of my marriage but I managed to pull through. Thankfully, I have now been well for four years. I have found keeping active is helpful, along with eliminating stressors that cause conflict, particularly with family members. I get great support from my friends and neighbours and appreciate every positive gesture, like being invited round to a friend's house for coffee. I have learned to grow as a person because of my mental health problems. In fact, I think my experiences in hospital have made me into a more helpful, understanding and knowledgeable person. Having said that, I also know the medication has made me forgetful and probably has depleted my brain cells. I haven't the learning capacity that I had twenty years ago and as such I am less intelligent than I used to be.

Finally, I would like to advocate that not everyone with bipolar leads dysfunctional lives, which is an opinion often formed when people listen to celebrities with the condition who have sold their stories for large amounts of cash, sensationalising their lives in the media. Even at my worst, I have never broken the law, defaulted on a loan or mortgage payment, never overspent and have never neglected or abused my child. I value health, education, and am a reliable and respected member of my community. But more importantly, I have become content with who I am.

Shane

Many find bipolar intolerable, yet tolerable when stable. They think when they're ill they will never recover – but then they get better and get on with life it's like they had never being unwell. Some say it is a vicious circle, fighting to become stable and then in a single day their world can come crashing down again without warning. Others find it empowering because without bipolar they feel they might have settled for lifestyles and/or relationships that weren›t right for them. Some have experienced frustration at not being able to do certain things, for example joining the armed forces, police or nursing, which adds to the stigma of being turned down for jobs. There are those who have formed lasting friendships, stating they met wonderful people through bipolar social networking sites. Here they share a bond, and although they will never meet 'in real life', realise the therapeutic value of sharing feelings with like-minded friends via telephone calls and email. Others become irritated when they overhear ignorant remarks in public or see negative things in the media. However, there are those who consider it human to say these things and say if they hadn't had bipolar they would probably throw words like 'nutter' and 'crazy' around too. Worry too comes into the frame and although some don't believe there's a

genetic link, they wonder if their behaviour, when
unwell, will affect their children and 'make' them
develop the condition too. Finally, bipolar for some is
the constant stress of taking medication, knowing it
is ruining their health and shortening their lives and
ultimately knowing its unfairness is never-ending.

I used to work fourteen-hour shifts, including some Saturdays, at a legal firm in the city. I pushed myself through sheer exhaustion to get through the high volume of work that arrived daily on my desk. My boss never asked me how I was managing. There was never an acknowledgement that we were short-staffed or over-stretched: instead she sent me endless demanding emails. Despite the long hours, the work still piled up. I started making mistakes, lacked concentration but just blamed it on tiredness. I didn't want my boss to think I couldn't handle pressure, so I disguised my true feelings and carried on everyday as if nothing was wrong.

My girlfriend at the time became pregnant. Initially, the news meant great joy to us. I was looking forward to becoming a father, but early on in the pregnancy she began to express doubts about whether it was the right time to have a baby. Then suddenly the rug was pulled from underneath my feet when she had an abortion without discussing it with me properly. I felt betrayed and when I confronted her, she shocked me more than anyone else had ever done before when she told me, almost cavalierly, that she had been raped before we met and couldn't bear thinking about the pain of childbirth because of the pain she had previously endured. Despite her disregard about my feelings towards our aborted baby, her story of rape upset me deeply and I reached out to her, comforted her and wanted her to believe she was safe with me and that no further harm would ever come to her. I wanted to be her protector, her sanctuary, her haven for safety and reassurance but instead, every time I made love to her, I felt nothing but guilt. Guilty that I was a man, and over time I became convinced that no matter how gentle I was with her during sex, that she would think of me as a rapist.

Depression descended me on like the darkness after a sunset. Beforehand, it was just stress but now I was starting to feel a sense of detachment. Enjoyment was being sucked out of me, like a plughole gurgling the remaining droplets of water down its drain. Nothing interested me anymore. It was like being in a dark place, a room where the sound of people making conversation was muffled. My GP prescribed antidepressants. Shortly afterwards I left my job because I could no longer stand the pressure. I also split up with my girlfriend. The love between us was eaten up by the realisation that neither of us were the same people we were when we first met. The tablets helped a bit, and although my senses were a little dulled, I felt enthusiastic enough to take a friend up on an offer of going travelling with him. Our destination was New Zealand, but firstly we stopped off in Thailand, where new faces and new experiences greeted me. Freedom from the turmoil I left behind in Britain automatically made me feel better. It was like a harness had been removed from my back after I stopped taking the medication.

Since adolescence I'd had a deep yearning to learn about the mysteries of the universe. In Thailand, I visited Buddhist temples and developed a keen interest in reincarnation. There I was able to reconnect with imprints from my previous lives. I had first started thinking about the role humans played in the universe when I was seven but with the new realisation of reincarnation and the belief that I had lived many times before came the realisation that humans are a little like recycled atoms. Someone gave me a book written by the Dalai Lama, which enriched my knowledge even further with his teachings on humility and peace. I enjoyed my time in Thailand even more because of the way it taught me to relax. My mind was at rest, like the calmness that follows a storm, making me feel well and happy.

From Thailand, my friend and I travelled on to New Zealand where I continued my interest in Buddhism. I went to various meetings, made new friends and began to acquire new optimism towards life by developing a newfound compassionate and openhearted approach to my future. My friend and I visited friends of his who lived in a boathouse. They lived a bohemian lifestyle, free from the trappings of wanting to be like other people. They loved living life close to the sea and felt in tune with their natural surroundings. I appreciated their philosophies and grew to respect the simplicity that life brings with less emotional and material baggage.

It was towards the end of my time in New Zealand when I began to become unwell, although neither I nor those in my company were aware of it or recognised what was happening. One day I was lying down sunbathing on the boardwalk that led to the boat, when suddenly I noticed that the timber beneath me began to disappear and when the last plank had vanished, I was left lying on the water. Jesus had created a miracle by walking on the water unaided and here I was lying on the water, floating in a similar surreal sense. This, too, felt like a miracle. Then I looked towards the surrounding mountains and trees. They too, one by one began to disappear. Next, the water from the marina began to drain from underneath me, inch by inch, until it left me lying on the bare sand dune. My body had gone from being physical to a pure energy force in a matter of minutes, leaving me with a feeling of total euphoria. I construed what was happening as a conversation taking place within me. I silently kept saying to myself, "I can free myself," and then out loud to those around me, "We can free ourselves." I remember having total sensation in my body, but also realising that I had the ability to become free of pain at any time I chose, so convincing was my new found state of being. The greatness and power of this feeling has never left me. Neither has the realisation that I don't need all the materialistic trappings that our consumer society convinces us we need. The true source of fortune is within our soul, how we feel and react, how we treat others and how we give gratitude to our higher being for the kindness of his blessings, no matter how small these may be.

After returning home to Britain, my spiritual quest continued but I wanted more people than myself to experience this freedom and began to spread the good news – "We can free ourselves" – to anyone who would listen. My family and friends became concerned about my behaviour but I was oblivious to their feelings. I began to visualise a light coming out of me and interpreted this as a sign that I could heal and open up peoples' consciousness. The thoughts in my head were comparable to the video clip of *Bohemian Rhapsody* by Queen, when several heads spiral around and eventually form into one. This is what sleep deprivation achieved. In hindsight, I can see why people thought I was crazy. My next memory after this was waking up in hospital several days later after having been hospitalised, tranquillised and placed under Section 2 of The Mental Health Act. I remained there for four weeks before being discharged and was prescribed Olanzapine to quell my mania. I remained on the medication for a few weeks but once I felt better, I stopped taking it. I resumed normal life once more and gradually felt well enough to look for a new job.

Six years passed between that manic episode and the next. During that period, I met my wife and became a practicing Buddhist. Life was good to me during those years. I liked my job, bought a house and some land and my wife and I planned for a baby. Indeed, all was going well until the birth of our son. My wife had a difficult pregnancy, which put pressure on us both, combined with everyday worries about work and money. Not eating or sleeping properly came to a climax when my wife was in hospital giving birth. In the UK, little thought is ever given to fathers of aborted babies – and not enough when babies are born. During the week of my son's birth I spent most of the time at the hospital, often not sleeping for seventy-two hours at a time. There wasn't a provision available in the hospital where fathers-to-be or new fathers could sleep for a few hours. So once again, I carried on like a car whose fuel tank was running dangerously low, until it came to a complete halt. A short hospitalisation followed, similar to the one I described earlier. The only difference was that I remained on medication for longer this time, but eventually weaned myself off it completely six months later.

I believe the cure for bipolar is within every person. I found mine through my faith. Buddhism opened and changed my mind about the world. I have discovered something that feels like a more normal state of being for me. I meditate on a daily basis because I know that change can only come from inside. People have to find that space, that connection to our true life source in order to develop the desire to change. As well as having developed this solid belief system, my wife and I farm our plot of land with great passion. I have a connection with the land and love planting trees, sowing vegetables and watching them grow. I eat healthily – lots of raw, wholesome food and fresh fruit smoothies from the fruit grown in our orchard. Most people go through periods of worrying about the meaning of life. I certainly spent most of my earlier life worrying about materialism, right up to the point when I came to despise it. Now I live life in a way that I feel is at ease with those around me. I am grateful for all the small beauties it holds, but ultimately I'm filled with astonishment and gratitude that I'm actually alive at all.

What being a carer means to me:

1. Being terrified
2. Trying to maintain my own sanity
3. Coping with terrible financial difficulties
4. Neighbours and friends telling me something they know nothing about
5. Many sleepless nights
6. Building up the courage to challenge the doctors
7. Feeling nervous
8. Being unable to reason with my daughter
9. Turning to alcohol for comfort
10. Despair.

Shelia

Jessica

I grew up in an inner city, where block after block of grey, drab-looking flats, daubed with graffiti, provided the scenery to any outsider brave enough to venture in. Vandalised telephone boxes and metal shutters on shop fronts ensured few strangers walked our streets – and those who did were looked on with suspicion, as they were usually social workers, bailiffs or the police. Clothes lines packed with washing hung from every balcony and obstructed views from both the outside and inside but thankfully concealed windows and front doors that had pieces missing. My parents were on the dole, with unemployment the norm in our part of the city. Traditionally, work on the nearby docks had provided employment, but the arrival of containerisation in the late eighties led to my father and hundreds like him losing their jobs. Then there were drugs, with daily sightings of syringes on the grass verges during the heroin epidemic of the eighties and early nineties, resulting in several drug addicts contracting AIDS. Gang-related drug-turf fights broke out between local thugs for the monopoly on drugs and cash, leading to many murders. Muggings were so common that many people didn't bother reporting them to the police because they thought their crime wouldn't be taken seriously, or feared reprisal from the perpetrator, who they often knew by name. Life played itself out like this daily and you either ended up oblivious to its misery or worst still – indifferent to it all.

It is hardly surprising I've had traits of melancholy in me since an early age, having grown up in such a depressing environment. The gloom and apathy got under my skin and somehow inside me, like dirt gets under your nails and buries itself in tiny crevices invisible to the human eye. I wanted to deal with my unhappiness better, but all I heard from those around me were stories that contained no hope about the economy, job losses, drugs and emigration. I was only eighteen and in a bad place as I listened to their spiel. I hated the way I felt, I couldn't understand it and hadn't the words or courage to tell anyone exactly how I felt. My family constantly asked, "Why are you like this?" And afterwards, when I spent increased periods in bed, their questions became more accusatory, implying, "Something must have happened to you to be like this." But nothing had happened. I was just like a thermometer whose temperature was permanently low and there was nothing within my control that I could do about it.

After completing secondary school I was lucky to get a job at a large supermarket. I didn't enjoy it but I saw it as a means of saving enough money to go on my first overseas holiday with friends. Then, a colleague, who was a similar age to me, suddenly died. This affected me in a strange way because although I wasn't close to the girl, her death made me start thinking about dying and the afterlife, bringing me to tears at the slightest thought of it. To make matters worse I was asked to take over her job, leaving me feeling haunted by her presence. I was also pestered by thoughts that I too was going to die young, and I couldn't sleep properly – resulting in me becoming so exhausted that I gave up working. But this then meant that I did not have enough money to go on holiday. Disgruntled friends deserted me as I was unable to put my feelings into words and tell them what was going on inside my head.

My mother took me to the GP, who prescribed antidepressants, but I stopped taking them after a few weeks because, if anything, they made me constantly drowsy but didn't ease my depression. My family found it difficult to understand me and often lost patience with me I felt pressurised, and although I felt drained of motivation I eventually got another job, this time in a department store. This was just to keep the peace at home, but shortly afterwards something extraordinary happened. The mercury in the thermometer began to rise, slowly at first and then rather fiercely. My personality became comparable to the weather and went from dull and cloudy to sunny with a gentle breeze. I became a party girl and started going to pubs, nightclubs, and house parties night after night. You could find me anywhere where there was alcohol and the promise of a good time. My confidence surged, allowing me to talk to strangers with a degree of newfound enthusiasm. I'm a lesbian but now I found myself sleeping with men, which left me feeling very confused and wondering if I was bisexual. But little did I know back then that my thermometer had erupted and there was no stopping me for another three months until it plummeted with a vengeance, ending with me waking up in a psychiatric hospital, without remembering how I had got there.

During my first hospitalisation I thought everyone was part of a pact to kill me. I suspiciously watched patients huddle in small groups, imaging they were whispering about me, convinced this was part of the scheme to have me murdered. When I saw psychiatrists and nurses in the office with the door closed, I interpreted this as a covert sign that a plan was being hatched for my demise because they too must hate me and, like the patients, must want me dead. The relief experienced at being discharged was incredible, because the air outside had never smelt so fresh. On the other hand, being manic can entail portraying the world as a beautiful place where you think anything is possible because three years later, when I was hospitalised again, I was convinced that I was a film-star and that everyone in the hospital – patients, doctors, nurses, domestic staff – were all part of the film crew. When I was young I loved watching old films and particularly loved Elizabeth Taylor in *Cleopatra*, which lingered in my mind. And now there I was, the star of a film that would rival my childhood idol. I imagined a life of grandeur where I'd never have to work in retail again. Instead, people would queue for my autograph and billboards showing my photo would appear all over the world, while I would earn a fortune in the process. I became suspicious of some of the patients though, and wondered if it was their ploy to stand next to me so that they could get their faces on camera. Or perhaps they were jealous of me, resentful that it was me who was the star, while they were just menial film assistants?

As the psychosis lessened, so too did the fantasy, and then one day I woke up and realised that I wasn't a star after all – just an ordinary person like the rest of the patients. After that, hospital was no longer enjoyable because my dreams of fame and riches were over. This was never more realised than when a nurse, who I had previously regarded as my director, walked up and handed me a little plastic tub containing Lithium and my antidepressants. It was like she was the film's director who had shouted "Cut!" after spotting a flaw, waking me to the real world, and in the absence of any dream to sustain me against this harshness, my heart sank low, making the rest of my stay long and monotonous.

Secrecy is sometimes necessary in life – but it is also a burden to carry. Last year, I decided to tell the truth about being bipolar to my manager, something I had hidden from all my previous employers. She was very understanding and I can now tell her when I have appointments at the clinic for Lithium blood level tests or when I have to see my psychiatrist. It's a relief not having to lie with a silly excuse when concealing information too difficult or embarrassing to reveal – which has made me feel freer. Admittedly, there are one or two inquisitive colleagues who suspected I had a medical condition and who had asked me what had been wrong with me. I felt a tiny bit awkward telling them the truth to satisfy their curiosity, but it was better than lying. Maybe they understand me better now and recognise that my condition brings difficulties, such as the exhaustion sometimes brought on by Citalopram or– the Lithium that sometimes causes my right hand to shake.

Music to me is as powerful as poetry is to other people and has got me through some very tough times over the past fifteen years. To me, it is a healer and contemplative. I often light some scented candles, lie on the couch and close my eyes as I absorb the words of a song. This is also a good way to visualise controlling stress and depression – it often becomes a case of mind over matter. There is a favourite affirmation I say to myself: *I am well and I am safe.* Aspects of how bipolar make me feel are exquisitely captured in the lyrics of the song *Everything's Not Lost* by Coldplay: ......*So if you ever feel neglected If you think that all is lost, I'll be counting up my demons, yeah. Hoping everything's not lost.........*

Friends helped me to decorate my flat when I moved in last year. It is a council flat but I have made it into a little palace. When I was in hospital I discovered that I was good at painting and it prompted me to take some evening classes in art. My modest creations from the course cover the walls of my flat. I now live with my Jack Russell but one day I hope to meet someone special and fall in love.

I find that the more I understand my illness, the easier it is to control. I don't think I can have power over it entirely, but I believe it is important to read the signs and withdraw when my mania, with its unpredictable behaviour, becomes unsettling to others and myself. My family are good people but they are not perfect. I have accepted this in the same way that I have accepted that I am not perfect, by developing enough resilience to handle confrontation. This helps, by being easy on them as well as myself. I try to help my mind to heal as much as possible, rather than mask it with medication – and this includes having a regular routine with sleep and eating a fairly balanced diet. Don't misinterpret me and think I am constantly watching my lifestyle and diet. I'm not, because I still smoke, but I have cut down on drinking wine. I am fully aware and accepting that life goes on regardless – and whatever calamity I experience, I know there are others who will have had to deal with far greater problems. I am grateful that my life isn't so bleak at the moment, and that my problems are kept to a minimum.

Michael

Every person has three lives. The outward life people see – the one you share with family and friends, the one you give your own personal account about. Then there is the life that is hidden – your past hidden from view, full of secrets that are not obvious. This is the life I chose not to entirely tell Declan Henry about because I felt shame. Then there's your inner life, the one that ticks away inside – comprising of dreams, hopes, aspirations and fantasies. This life is private.

I loved building model aircrafts when I was a young boy and had several hundred kits, ranging from the F4 Phantom, English Electric Lightning, Hunter and Canberra models to an F104 Star fighter and Darken sets. During my youth, most children I knew could name every model of car, while I could identify most aircraft. Happy memories came flooding back when my sister took me to a military display in a museum. The outing allowed me to forget about my claim for incapacity benefit. This is playing on my mind because I dread receiving a letter instructing me to attend an interview to explain my circumstances. It is not that I have anything to hide or mind answering personal questions. It is the approach these officials take when dealing with claimants, subjecting you to a slow and cold interrogation because they are convinced you are lying and feel it's their duty to ooze out shame and guilt when you ask for money they feel isn't your entitlement.

I hate living on benefits because I'd worked all my life until that fateful day. There can be no conceivable explanation other than him having pure evil in his heart, for him to have expressed such putrid hatred. He was simply a psychopath, because his cold-blooded callousness was immune to the suffering it inflicted upon his victims that afternoon, when he set off to Brixton with a nail bomb in his rucksack. David Copeland, later to become known as the 'London nail bomber,' aimed his attacks at London's black, Bangladeshi and gay communities. The first attack was on Saturday 17th April 1999, in Brixton. The bomb was taped inside a sports bag and contained explosives from fireworks, which Copeland primed and planted outside a supermarket. I had worked in the hospital as a porter for ten years and seen appalling injuries including gunshot and stab wounds, but nothing prepared me for the sights of that night. Fifty people were seriously injured because of the four-inch nails that Copeland had packed around the bomb. I still vividly recall the panic, screams and grief when the wounded and dead were wheeled in, one after the other. A man had half his face blown off by the force of the explosion. There was a woman who came in with nails ingrained into her head. One of the nails was within a millimetre of her brain; her CT scan showed that just another millimetre and she would have died. And then there was a six-week-old baby with nails embedded into her face and chest.

I'd followed in my father's footsteps and served my apprenticeship as a butcher. Early morning trips to Smithfield market meant being able to pick up the gear. I had a reliable dealer, both discreet and good with credit, although I was earning a decent wage at the time. I first took cocaine when I was nineteen and became hooked almost instantly. After work, the stinking overalls that smelt of blood and dead carcasses were replaced with crisp clothing from my collection of blue suits with velvet collars, matched with raised leopard skin design shoes, black shades and a generous coating of Brylcreem that doubled as cologne. I loved the kudos of being a teddy boy. I loved the laddish company that came with being this cult figure. No one dared mess with my gang of friends from South East London. We stuck together and were like brothers who looked out for one another. Sometimes we got mixed up in violent fights between rival gangs but mainly we just hung out together and shared our gear because one of the golden rules was making sure your mates never went short.

My bipolar started a few months after the bombing, with flashbacks of bodies torn apart – and accompanied by high bursts of energy, making me feel like I was constantly running late for something and needed to rush in the process. In order to stabilise my moods, my psychiatrist prescribed Sodium Valproate along with Olanzepine, which unfortunately led me to develop a large paunch. I was also given antidepressants – and a beta-blocker for panic attacks which continue to blight my life. It's the physical side of these that is most nasty. A knotted pain develops in my stomach.

I know instantly what is going to happen next because my adrenaline slips, draining my flow of oxygen and my stomach muscles ache so badly that it causes spasms. Sweat pours out of my body, wanting me to retch, but I am unable to vomit. These attacks last thirty to forty minutes until the feeling of panic subsides and I return to normal. The most dreaded fear of all is when I have to go outdoors. I've experienced panic attacks on buses and in busy shops. It is a living hell being surrounded by strangers who stop and stare as the sweat drips from my brow – and all I want is for my lungs to fill with air so that I can breathe easily again. So when this happens I return home immediately, because I know the attack won't stop until I am back indoors and begin to feel safe again.

Even with antidepressants I get depressed, and when this happens I'll stay in bed for days with my body feeling trapped under the duvet, making me unable to move, as if I have been tied up with a strong rope. I compare times like this to being in the theatre. When the show ends and the curtain comes down, I'm alone and the auditorium is dark, making me feel so depressed that I verge on being suicidal. "Please God, I never will do this." As well as not eating, I don't wash, the house becomes neglected. I can't read. I can't concentrate. Then the depression eases off. It goes away by itself. The lights come on. The curtain begins to rise and the show starts once more. I resume enthusiasm for reading again, mainly biographies, military and nature stories. I watch westerns and documentaries on television. I love animals, particularly cats because they never harm humans. So I lavish attention on the three I've got, fearing they've been neglected while their master was ill. I am blessed in the sense that I have a good family network and good neighbours who keep an eye out for me.

Ah, those were some of the best days of my life. I met a nice girl in my twenties and got married and had a son. My father-in-law set me up in business – a large shop with a flat overhead. Money flowed in during the 1970s but greed led to mistakes and the biggest one of all was to sell the business. I thought I was invincible after the bank made a silly error by putting double the amount of money from the sale of the business into my account. I kept my mouth shut and went to start a new life in Spain. A new business venture in a nightclub took my interest. It wasn't long before every night became a party with lots of booze, cocaine and prostitutes. But then the business began to falter and not long afterwards I was arrested at Heathrow for fraud for not declaring the bank's error. Bankruptcy and prison quickly followed. All my money had been squandered, my wife left me after I was imprisoned – leaving me a broken man. She didn't want to know me after I was released from prison and forbade me contact with my son. I really wanted to be the best father in the world to him. My own dad died when I was young, leaving my mother and sister to bring me up. Although I stopped taking cocaine, I took up drinking Special Brew lager instead. I knew it disagreed with me, but that didn't deter me from drinking it. I used to imagine people were looking at me after I'd drunk a few cans and challenge them, often expressing racist, abusive views in the process. Afterwards, I'd hate myself but the cycle of self-loathing would only last a few days until the next dole cheque, the next drinking spree and again I'd shout and be aggressive to whoever crossed my path. Perhaps this made me blank out the thoughts I had of becoming the outcast of the family – until I landed on my feet again when I got the porter's job.

Since the bombing, I have adapted a hard approach towards life, to the point where I am now insensitive at times. I cannot bear to listen to people whinging about minor problems. Coping with depression and mood swings is a full-time job, but if I could achieve total cessation of these debilitating panic attacks, then I might be able to see light at the end of the tunnel. I am waiting for some more counselling, because I found previous sessions beneficial. Talking openly and frankly about my emotions is a good way of learning why I lean towards pessimism over optimism. Indeed, I feel if I hadn't received previous support from my counsellor or if I weren't on my present medication, I would be dead by now.

What does the future hold? For the moment I feel like I am playing in a football match but my fitness levels are under par. It is half-time and the other team are winning. I am in the dressing room, sweating, breathless and my body aches. I listen to the coach barking his criticisms, berating me and the other players for our poor performance. He calls us useless and lazy, pointing out our mistakes and reminding us that if we don't improve in the second half, we will lose the match. I feel guilty and ashamed, but am determined to go back onto the pitch with renewed vigour and play much better than in the first half. I want to score lots of goals and win the game.

I am now in my early sixties and want good health again – as well as happiness and freedom from the emotional pain of recent times, as I enter into the autumn phase of my life. I want to be free of bipolar before it beats me. I don't know how I'm going to do this, but that's my wish anyway. People wish for things all the time and some get lucky. That's what wishes are for. They are there for everyone and I've earmarked what I would most like to come true for me.

Bipolar and me means:

1. Living with a fear of debilitation
2. Constant uncertainty
3. Feeling ashamed
4. Desiring to feel comfortable in my own skin
5. Being spiritual
6. Wanting to share with others how I am feeling
7. The necessity of having to challenge malign and uncaring people in authority
8. Anxious that people won't listen to me when I'm unwell
9. Getting up to urinate every two hours during the night. Anyone got a nappy?
10. If I think the shakes are bad now – what will they be like when I'm 64?!

Thomas

Rebecca

"I am excessively slothful, and wonderfully industrious by fits. There are epochs when any kind of mental exercise is torture, and when nothing yields me pleasure but the solitary communion with the 'mountains & the woods' – the 'altars' of Byron. I have thus rambled and dreamed away whole months, and awake, at last, to a sort of mania for composition. Then I scribble all day, and read all night, so long as the disease endures."

Edgar Allen Poe

Does bipolar run in my family? Now, that is a question I would like answered. My grandparents left Ireland for a new life in England in the 1950s but sadly their future turned out differently than they had intended. My grandmother went out and spent the money they had saved for a house on shoes, hats and new outfits, resulting in them having to live in a council property instead. She was considered extravagant – someone who wasn't good with money. She died when I was very young and few people now ever mention her name but I still think about her. She had a lovely smiling face. I once asked my father if he thought she had bipolar but he dismissed the idea before changing the conversation.

Having a manic episode is completely unlike a physical illness, where you take time out to recover and once well can resume normal life again. Mania is like a storm, but worse. It is like the aftermath of a riot, whereby effort is required to fix all the smashed windows and clean up the pieces of debris, piece by piece, street after street until the district has been put back to the way it was before the disturbance took place.

I had symptoms of bipolar before I was diagnosed at the age of twenty-three, consisting of severe anxiety and extremes of mood along with paranoia that noticeably affected my way of life before I started my career as a music teacher. I never had much confidence and feared public speaking, but regardless of this I went into teaching, which I always wanted to do, but believe the stress I put myself under caused my bipolar to spiral out of control. Indeed, my worst depression was when I was teaching and was signed off work for several months. I felt like a useless blob, worthless, and couldn't bring myself to get out of bed after routinely sleeping fifteen hours everyday. I was unable to eat and wash and no matter how messy the house became, I couldn't have cared less. I cried and wished I were dead. I felt like I had flu. I ached all over, I was completely withdrawn from friends and family, didn't even want to answer the phone. Then there were the hallucinations. I used to see people whose eyes glowed walking around the house as well as imagining there were wasps crawling across my face. All of those experiences felt so real to me. I remember feeling very scared all the time and heard that people on drugs experience similar things, but I definitely wasn't on drugs.

My worst manic episode was when I was on anti-depressants. I handed in my notice after deciding I no longer wanted to teach. I wanted this to be a fresh beginning – a new life away from my old one, so I changed telephone numbers, deleted former friends and work colleagues from Facebook and avoided talking to any of them when we met in public. My boyfriend and I then nearly lost our home because I had spent all our money and got myself into a world of debt, culminating in several county court judgements. I then started to plan for us to move away and arranged to move into three different places all at the same time. I wasn't eating or sleeping, I was hearing voices and my night terrors, when I did sleep, were pretty horrific.

It wasn't planned and nobody expected it to happen, least of all me. But no excuse could remedy the shame I felt after I overdosed on antidepressants. I also discovered that a suicide attempt did not solve my debts, nor did it prevent loads of guilt as a result of my crazy spending. My boyfriend was deeply upset by my actions, but then he always seems to get the raw end of the deal. I am just lucky that he understands me because when I'm unwell I am prone to saying something brutally insensitive or insulting. He's been told he's a *shit* boyfriend and that it was his fault I tried to kill myself and that his Dad, who is dead, would be ashamed of him. Friends too have suffered with outbursts from my vulgar tongue – I once casually remarked to my best friend that I thought her husband was fat and useless. After these eruptions I am guilt-ridden, but at the time I have no control over them as they explode so naturally when I'm angry, frustrated or in an agitated mood.

When I was young, the only person who I felt took the time to understand what I was trying to say was my grandfather. I was always overly emotional and excitable as a child and I suppose as an adult I still am. My grandfather passed away when I was nine years old and it wasn't until

I met my boyfriend that I really opened up to someone because of profound shyness. My parents were aware of my self-confidence issues and my mother once bought me a Paul McKenna hypnosis tape, which seemed to help. I have often wondered, especially after researching bipolar, if I brought it on myself. I have come to the conclusion that because of my lack of confidence and by forcing myself to be confident in situations at work that caused me anxiety, I may have inadvertently placed too much pressure on my brain.

Some people trivialise depression – often unintentionally by dropping a trite remark on a depressed person as if was something they needed to hear. While these thoughts help in a handful of cases, they won't cure the masses of depression. I have found a list of things that people should be mindful of not saying to someone with bipolar because, personally, I find them patronising and belittling. I've also added a few of the awful things people have said to me over the years as well.

"It's all in your mind."

"Be Strong."

"Stop feeling sorry for yourself."

"There are a lot of people worse off than you."

"You have nothing to be unhappy about."

"Cheer up."

"You should get off all those pills."

"Most folks are about as happy as they make up their minds to be."

"Get a job."

"You don't 'look' depressed."

"You're just looking for attention."

"Everybody has a bad day now and then."

"Why don't you smile more?"

"A person your age should be having the time of their life."

"The only one you're hurting is yourself."

"You can do anything you want if you just set your mind to it."

"You brought this on yourself."

"Get off your rear and do something."

"Snap out of it."

"Just try a little harder."

"I know how you feel – I was depressed once for several days."

"You don't like feeling that way? So change it."

"You're a real downer to be around."

"You are embarrassing me."

"You're dragging me down with you."

"You're just being immature."

"You are your own worst enemy."

"That is life – get used to it."

"Life is full of ups and downs!"

I am me and I won't change myself for anyone! I now realise that my life is not all bad because I only have to take a step back and see the love and support I get from my boyfriend, family and friends to know that. I am trying to take better care of myself and in order to avoid stress, I have not returned to teaching. Basically, I am taking time out to decide what I want to do in the long-term future. I read a lot and draw as I've always been creative, and find this outlet very therapeutic. I also do voluntary work looking after an elderly man in my neighbourhood. He is a gentle soul, who makes me smile as he reminds me of my grandfather. I take multi-vitamins and fish oils (I have read that fish oils can act as a natural mood stabiliser). I also try my best to stick to the medication prescribed. I cycle everywhere and always make sure I have something to look forward to everyday. This may be preparing a nice dinner for my boyfriend and I, going shopping or to the cinema, starting a new painting or illustration, reading a new book or just meeting up with a friend for a drink and chat.

Kevin

I hadn't realised my appreciation or understood the depth of our friendship until he died. I missed him terribly, but over time I began to question what secret he was harbouring – what person or thing had wounded him so deeply that he thought death was its only answer. I kept questioning why he was unable to trust me. Having his death thrust upon me, I had no idea how to process the grief. My psychiatrist later told me what happened was a *spiritual emergency*. His philosophy was that a breakdown was a *breakthrough* where otherwise, had a crisis not occurred, personal growth wouldn't have been able to take place. But this wasn't before I endured months of going from being an ordinary school teacher – a normal and straightforward man – to someone who developed grandiose ideas about my job, was unable to sleep for three to four days at a time and became so exhausted I started imagining my dead friend's shadow was standing at the back of the classroom, until I finally collapsed with grief.

My psychiatrist prescribed Valium, which calmed me down and made me sleep almost continuously for a week. I had no idea what a remarkable man he was until I read his name in a newspaper article. I am talking about the late Dr Michael Corry*, who became my psychiatrist and remained so for nine years up until his untimely death in 2010. Dr Corry always maintained that many of the leading psychiatrists do not have basic counselling skills. When I met Dr Corry he immediately empathised with the bipolar state I was in, he clearly knew its territory, and he treated my fragile emotional state with compassion. His health plan was to keep me away from psychiatric hospitals and institutions. He saw a use for conventional medicine but in a controlled way, to be used in emergencies for a short time only.

Dr Corry also insisted that I have psychotherapy, with the aim of me gaining insight into my bipolar and to emotionally move on from the death of my friend. During these sessions, I unburdened my troubles to the counsellor, telling her that I had let my friend down and was to blame for his suicide. I described to her how this torturous and unwelcome thought had taken up residency in my consciousness and appeared to have no intention of moving. My counsellor had a spiritual slant to her thinking and spoke of soul healing. She put me in touch with an American clairvoyant who was in the country twice yearly. I immensely enjoyed the readings and although I kept an open mind, I was led to wonder if the reason behind my sudden, irrational manic behaviour was attributed to an energy blockage from a past life where I had unresolved issues. This wasn't a possibility I could discuss with my staunch Catholic family because I knew they would rebuff such an idea as spiritual mumbo jumbo. They were firm in their belief that a person has only one lifetime here on earth – and that when he or she dies, they go to either heaven or hell depending on how well they lived their life.

I also went to see a homeopath for treatment. It's hard to quantify how I benefited from homeopathy but I know I always felt better afterwards. The appointments usually lasted three quarters of an hour and gave me the opportunity to speak about my feelings, relationships and how things were going for me generally. I know there is much debate about homeopathy within certain parts of the medical establishment, but my own view is that an open mind is a good thing and I know that over the years being able to confide in my homeopath has helped me grow and mature, and that had I not sought this help I wouldn't be as wise about things as I am now.

I managed to stay well for several years until I crumbled under intense pressure from a bullying headmaster and a demanding management board. I worried that my teaching style wasn't good enough and that my students would fail their exams. I endeavoured to work harder and teach better. Although elation feels great, anyone who experiences it knows the sensation isn't normal. Before it occurs, you have a feeling that something is building up in the background but there is never enough time to do anything about it because next thing, you are elated. The feeling is like being at a party with flashing lights and images where the music is loud and you are loud with it. But the reality is that you are vulnerable, like a teenager that needs mothering. Elation takes away from you things that you love. I have always enjoyed drama and getting into character but this requires concentration and preparation. Mania does not allow this because it eats you up and saps your energy. I know the feeling only too well. I was once doing a rehearsal for a Christmas concert when I became so immersed in concentration that something clicked inside my head, making me realise I was in the throes of a manic episode. With this I took myself off to hospital.

This was the first time in my life that I became accustomed to a routine of being drugged. Unfortunately,

Dr Corry had died the previous year and I was then under a new psychiatrist – who was totally authoritative and medication-driven and left me with the feeling that she was talking down to me. It would be impossible for there to be a greater contrast between Dr Corry's approach and hers. She believed that people with bipolar were flawed and chemically imbalanced and that drug treatment was the only answer in addressing this problem. My mood plummeted whilst in hospital, sinking me into a dark depression. My medication was increased from 300mg Seroquel to 800mg and I was also prescribed Sodium Valproate to prevent fluctuations in mood. My psychiatrist casually dropped into the conversation during a ward round that I had been "Footsteps away from having ECT treatment." I knew little about ECT and looked it up on the internet. The only word that sums my thoughts up on this is hate. I shudder at the thought of how that woman even considered the appropriateness of this treatment. It fills me with dread as to how this treatment would have wiped out large chunks of my memory, how precious images of my childhood would have been lost without a moment's hesitation, in the same way that photographs get irrevocably lost when a virus attacks the hard drive of a computer. The loss would be immeasurable and I thank God this did not happen.

Medication makes me feel restricted and I feel less of a man because of my condition. I feel insignificant in front of other people. This feeling often leads into a land of darkness. I call these my *black down days*. It doesn't help having to go to an outpatient clinic where I see people looking physically wrecked from taking medication. I look around at the facial features and mannerisms. There is never a trace of real joy in sight, with any minor sign of happiness artificially induced. Human contact is important at these times but when I'm depressed I find it hard to talk to family and friends. I don't have many friends but with the few I have I like to keep the company fresh. I don't want to appear needy and like to have everyday conversation and amusement rather than focus on me and my woes. When I'm lonely, I often ring the Samaritans. A friendly voice at the other end of the line brings reassurance that there is someone willing to listen. I also write letters to them because I find it a release to write my feelings down on paper. Getting a response isn't important.

But the positive thing about depression is that you are forced to learn about yourself during the solitary moments. Dr Corry always told me that depression is an emotion – not a disease. Knowing this doesn't stop me looking for meaning in my life. Nor does it stop me making sense out of it. I'm 42 now. I question what I have achieved over the last two decades. There are days when I close the curtains in my sitting room and ponder about the answer to this question. Maybe I'll return to teaching one day, or perhaps I'll seek another occupation that is less stressful. I believe bipolar is only part of a bigger picture because my psychotherapist once drew me a pie chart and divided out the various sections of my life to see where bipolar came into the equation. I clearly saw it was only a part of me and not the defining component that dominates my existence. Are these easy words to say or do I really believe them? When I'm low I do not see my worth or place in life and I shy away from human contact. But the irony is that what I am shying away from is exactly what I crave and need. I would love to have a close friend who has chosen to be with me and for us to love each other. We would talk, laugh and dance together. He would be someone who would understand my bipolar and offer me support and compassion. How I long for someone like that to be in my life.

* The late Dr Michael Corry (1948-2010) was the founder of the Wellbeing Foundation, Ireland. He was a fearless campaigner for the rights of mental health service users and all those suffering psychological distress; an opponent of bio-psychiatry and its reliance on psycho-pharmacology and a staunch campaigner for the abolition of ECT.

When I'm well – I am:

1. Bright and happy
2. Kind
3. Energetic
4. Fun-loving
5. Intelligent
6. Warm and welcoming
7. Generous
8. A good listener
9. Peaceful
10. Responsible.

Jade

Joan

We met and married in London in the early seventies. He was handsome in his youth, tall and slim with lovely jet-black hair and a dimple. He was always laughing and loved telling jokes. We used to go to dances with other friends in Cricklewood and he loved having an audience to practice his latest joke on.

> *Have you heard the one about the man in the mental hospital? The psychiatrist asked the man what would happen if he cut off one of his ears. "I'd be blind in one eye," the man replied. The psychiatrist wrote down the answer before then asking, "What would happen if I cut off both your ears?" – "I'd be blind in both me eyes." "Why do you say that?" asked the psychiatrist – "Me cap'd fall down into me eyes."*

We decided to return home to help his widowed father farm his land. I didn't think back then that there was anything wrong with him. He went through mood swings in the early years of our marriage, but I thought these were a result of arguments he had had with his father. They were often like two children, squabbling over a toy because they always wanted to do little things differently on the farm.

Over time he became a slave to the land and his cattle, working from dawn to dusk. We weren't well off and relied heavily on the monthly creamery cheque. The stress was awful when he'd pace up and down the house shouting, arguing and getting aggressive at the slightest irritation. I threatened to leave. He threatened suicide. We reached a compromise when I found a job and, although a woman going to work in the rural community during this era was frowned upon, it proved to be my salvation. It was an escape from the mayhem and brought a little piece of normality into my life.

But chaos resumed every night when I returned home. He would be waiting for me like a fox outside a hen house. He would be washed, shaved and wearing a clean vest.

"Let me be nice to you," were his signalling words for sex, and he would repeat them over and over again.

He was like an animal, a predator constantly on heat in pursuit of its prey. His demands would continue until I had no other choice but to relent. I was often kept awake until three o'clock in the morning and then after a few hours sleep we both had to be up again. Another day, another chance for him to cause more wreckage. He never ate breakfast before going off to milk the cows. I'd be busy getting the children ready for school, making packed lunches, reminding them not to forget their books and getting myself dressed for work. I used to try to leave the house as quietly as possible, hoping he wouldn't notice. But the bastard had a scent for this type of thing and just as I'd open the door, he would be standing outside and before I'd be able to utter a word he would have said those immortal words, "Let me be nice to you." No matter how many times I refused, no matter how many times I told him to stop pestering me, he continued. He never forced himself upon me but it was a permanent fear, a permanent obstacle that made life unbearable because each time I had sex with him, it made me loathe him, and myself, that little bit more.

There were never enough hours in the day. Life was fast paced, mechanical, as if we were in frenzy – fearful that a storm was coming and we weren't prepared for its impact. I was often crying out for sleep. There was little rest at weekends after he had bought a car because he insisted on taking the children and me out on trips to various towns and seasides. There was little peace with the neighbours either, but there was one neighbour in particular whom he targeted. It was Brendan, a fellow farmer, a bachelor who lived in our village, who was often on the receiving end of his vulgar tongue. He held an unfathomable grudge towards him. I could never understand it because Brendan was a lovely quiet, decent, hardworking man who wouldn't harm a fly. If Brendan's cattle broke into one of our fields or vice versa, or if a stray animal appeared on the road, my husband, irrespective of the circumstances, would go to Brendan's house and at the top of his voice would summon him to come outside. He would then swear at him, using every profanity in the dictionary. I used to have to intervene or send one of our older children to calm him down, but he would usually refuse to stop until he had exhausted himself. This happened on several occasions, but the strange thing is that after every dispute, the next time he'd meet Brendan he would be friendly and chat to him like they were old friends. He even invited Brendan round a few times to play cards at our house, along with some other neighbours and friends. But he was conniving and spiteful and knew exactly how to humiliate someone, because on one of those occasions, during a game of poker, he turned to Brendan and said something completely unexpected:

"Now tell me Brendan, when was the last time you let air into a woman?"

It was utterly humiliating. I hung my head with embarrassment and after everyone had left, I laid into him.

"Don't you ever show me up like that again – how could you say such a thing to him, have you no shame?" But that was a silly question, because I knew he had no shame. He lost it, along with his self-respect, somewhere in his life, without realising they were gone.

He lay on his back and screamed "No!" His body shook before he squirmed from left to right. It was like he was in a tight space being followed by someone he feared but the only way out was to lie down and creep towards the exit by pushing his entire strength down into his legs, to make them go as fast as possible to escape. The heat from his body was intense, with droplets of sweat dripping from his forehead down onto his face. Then suddenly he would bolt upright in bed, open his eyes before laying down again and going back to sleep as if nothing had happened. Nightmares like this were repeated every couple of nights. I constantly told him about them but he used to laugh at me or say something flippant. "Aaarah, what are you talking about, I must have been just snoring."

I mentioned them to his sister once but she made light of them, saying he used to have them as a child – but I used to lay there beside him, wondering what was going on in his head. I would have given anything to have got inside his dreams.

I could feel the heat of the bull's breath on my back as I ran through the fields. I counted to a hundred as I took long strides through the meadows. Picking blackberries from the bramble had led me into this unfortunate situation, making me forget about the big black beast whose territory I had trespassed upon, uninvited and unwelcome. I had never run this fast before, never knew that my legs could carry me with such great speed as I raced towards the sanctuary of the hill. I knew there was a tree there I could climb, where I would be safe. Bulls are not boys. They're not as clever and they can't climb trees, you know? Next thing I was on top of the tree breathing a sigh of relief, looking down to jest my cleverness at outsmarting my enemy, who was now nowhere to be seen. Suddenly, I saw the leather belt. It too was black in colour with its buckle glistening in the sun, as he held it tightly in his hands. I couldn't bring myself to look at his face. Instead, I looked at my hands and discovered they were covered in blood – my blood.

Life struggled by until matters came to a climax. His father's sudden and unexpected death hit him hard. One day I walked into the kitchen and found him crying. At first they were terrifyingly big, heavy sobs, which eased off to a sniffling sound like a punctured tyre with the hissing sound of air escaping. He went to bed and stayed there for days before he started getting up for short periods. He became fearful of going outdoors and was content to leave the running of the farm to our eldest son, something that ordinarily he would never have allowed because he liked to be in control. But he wasn't in control any longer, and during meal times he just picked at his food. He hated noise and if the television was on it had to be switched off. Likewise with conversation. That too had to be kept to a minimum. We became a silent house. Nothing I said could shake him out of this and after a couple of days I decided to call the doctor. He was taken to a psychiatric hospital and diagnosed with *Manic Depression.*

Like him, I knew very little about this condition, and if I'm honest I had only heard it being spoken about on the radio once, but paid little attention to what was being said. But now my husband had it and it felt like it a mystery. But the doctors said it could be sorted with medication. After he came home from hospital he became secretive and ashamed that there was something wrong with him. Although he eventually stopped taking his medication, he never went back to his more exuberant ways. On the whole he appeared calmer and there were fewer demands for sex. But then for the next ten years he became the best symbol of a seesaw ever, because his periods of mania and depression constantly battled against each other. The arguments continued with Brendan. The sulks, fears and irritations remained in full flow, followed by depressive moments, sleepiness, silence and self-pity. He wouldn't allow me to attend his outpatient appointments with his psychiatrist because he knew that I would tell them the truth about what he was really like at home. I wrote a letter to his psychiatrist once, but didn't get a reply so I never bothered again.

Time passes quickly, years roll by and then the day arrives when you look in the mirror and see how aged you have become.

Our separation wasn't swift or abrupt. It happened gradually over time. After one of our eldest children left home, I could move into the spare bedroom. While drifting along with everyday humdrum, our lives shifted slowly away in different directions. He had his friends in the pub for company. He called them his drinking buddies. I referred to them as his cronies, the local misfits who hung out in the pub together and talked rubbish. I joined a local women's group, where I met new friends and joined in activities, including keep-fit classes and a book club. Socialising opened up new awareness in me, broadened my thinking and made me realise there was another world away from him and his problems. He started to collect junk from skips and the farm and house began to look like a scrap yard. Maybe his collecting of scrap was symbolic because I, too, felt like a piece of junk. Our son was taking good care of the farm, so there was less pressure on me in that respect. I knew he would never change. I knew I could never change the circumstances. So by the time I moved into rented accommodation our lives were so empty of each other that I suspect my absence wasn't noticed until days later.

I still see him occasionally. He'll come around and sit quietly in the corner and sometimes try to tell a joke:

"Have you heard the one about the man at the undertakers?"

The problem is I've heard them hundreds of times before and no longer find them funny.

If it weren't for my children, I sometimes think that I would have wasted my life. But If I'm honest, a tiny part of me still holds on to the happy memories I have of when we first met in London. I keep telling myself that he is not all bad and that I must have loved him once, but even the memories have become faded and exhausted. I keep my faith in God because I know He understands everything. My mother always said the rosary every night and I now too follow this tradition. I usually start with a Father Peyton* prayer asking that my husband's mind is healed and that he finds peace:

God, Our Father, your wisdom is displayed in all creation and the power of your grace is revealed in the lives of holy people, who inspire us to trust you more fully and to serve others more generously. In a unique way, you blessed the life and work of your servant Patrick Peyton, CSC, and made him a fervent apostle of Mary, Queen of the Holy Rosary and Mother of us all. Through his intercession, we ask for this favour...Please grant it, if it is for your honour and glory, through Christ our Lord. Amen.

There is nothing left I can do about it but pray. Life has turned out the way it has. I have to accept it for what it is. We are growing old now, not together – but apart. I see couples our age in town, looking happy and contented in their retirement. But my happiness has to be different to theirs and there is no good to be achieved by wallowing in self-pity. I have to face the future, whatever it may bring, but for now I am enjoying some well-earned peace. A little solace in the wake of the deluge of destruction that surrounded and consumed the best years of my life.

* Father Patrick Peyton (1909–1992) hailed from a family of nine in County Mayo before emigrating to America, where he was ordained a priest in 1941. After recovering from tuberculosis, he devoted his life to the Blessed Virgin Mary. Pope John Paul 11 officially opened his cause of beatification in 2001 and he now has the title 'Servant of God'.

Sean

Psychiatrists have very little time for the mentally insane, no time at all for the sane – no matter how mad they might be.

Freud

People attend church every Sunday and listen to stories about Jesus and his disciples having visions as contained within the gospel – without questioning for a second the sanity or logic of this. But the moment a person says he or she hears or sees something paranormal, a finger is wagged at them, suggesting they are mad, strange and need locking up.

I love going for walks in my beloved County Roscommon – close to Lough Key and the Forest Park, which is one of Ireland's principal lakeside parks set in 840 acres of prime land on the outskirts of Boyle. Here I have spent many hours of immense satisfaction exploring the estate's nature walks, ring-forts, bog-garden and its expansive grounds where deer wander freely, oblivious of their watching admirers. Here I ponder about people, places, my life and situations in general because I am a deep thinker. I developed a passion for reading in my late twenties – novels, poetry, history texts and books on eastern religions.

I have mixed feelings about my childhood. Some days I crave a return to this time when my sanity wasn't questioned and when I hadn't any worries. In those early days, I idolised my father. In my eyes, he was a giant amongst giants, someone to look up to and to emulate. Over time I became a replica of his character and personality. A friend wrote this poem, *Childhood Dreams*, in which the words capture my love for him.

There are times when loneliness
Is very strong within me
And alone I walk the shore
Where bright pebbles take me
Back to happy sun lit days
Where wine was drank at ease
And rushing something only
The city dwellers understood,
Powerful the calling of the waves,
As children tend to their sandcastles,
Left abandoned
As the ice cream bell calls
Little white feet to its happy door
And granny upon her deck chair
As mother graces her strong shoulders
With a shawl and daddy calls us
To his care, where once more
The cows await feeding
And milking our important highlight
Of the evening as down
The little road we take the churn
To the Knocknagreena river
To cool till the morning milkman comes

> *Back again from my happy dreams*
> *To sober thoughts and oft at night*
> *I cry in my sleep*
> *For a man who loved his children*
> *As a farmer loves his fields.*

My father may have secretly loved me and my family but his levels of brutality towards us were ever visible. By the time I reached my early twenties, I felt lost and abandoned. I no longer viewed him in such high esteem and had realised the folly of ever believing him to be a good man. With the mist over my perception now lifted, I questioned my purpose and place in the world. With this reality laid bare, I acknowledged the violence I witnessed with my drunken father regularly hitting my mother. Terror, brutality and witnessing violence were my childhood friends. They were also my teacher. Is it ever possible to reclaim a lost childhood? Seeing my father's behaviour resulted in me drinking from an early age, and resulted in me engaging in regular disputes and fights when my mind became fogged by alcohol. But still I was convinced that I belonged. This always begged the question though of *where* I belonged?

People were incarcerated there until they died while others committed suicide or mysteriously died with their deaths hushed up by the hospital to prevent scandal. It was more than a dreadful place. It was evil, and while places of its kind were constructed in both Ireland and England as a result of ignorance, the end result was the same – nobody ever left cured or alive. It had been a psychiatric hospital for several decades before it was closed and turned into a prison in the nineties. This large grey, drab building with bars on its windows couldn't be mistaken for anything other than what it was – an institution. It had also been a sanatorium in the 1940s for patients with tuberculosis – so altogether its interior was accustomed to ghoulish sights, misery and suffering. It wouldn't have been able to cope with anything else. I recall having an eerie sense of foreboding loneliness as I walked along its dark, cold corridors. Psychiatry in Ireland, like most places, is not geared up for therapeutic input. The patient is just given drugs to treat the presenting problem and, invariably, this turns into a lifetime's chore. Indeed, the problems that affected my mind never crept above the parapet. My suffering, my loneliness, my flashbacks, the reminders, my dreams, my scratched psyche were all ignored.

A piece of prose by my poet friend entitled *Tortured Minds* sums up the mire of my pain most adequately:

Scattered dreams and deep illusions, fantasy of a world that could not exist even in heaven, there is a deep past – and now a lonely present – with the future in the obscure. The drowning cry, I am sinking, going under, and the silent cry of help can only be heard in an era of deep understanding, more freedom of speech, less bitterness and within this mind the agony outweighs normality and the healing process takes countless dark days. The locked doors cannot frighten the strong minded but the weakness held deep within each individual is brought to the light and the guilty emotions are forever holding us

back, but are the least important thing in an already
tortured mind.

Did I belong in a psychiatric hospital, where I was given drugs to suppress my anger and numb my assumed insanity, or did I belong at home with my dysfunctional family and violent father – or in the rural community where I grew up with its people whispering unkind and judgmental thoughts behind my back? Or was it somewhere else in the world, away from my life, where I might belong but was unable, for whatever reason, to reach? The first time I was incarcerated in hospital I arrived with one of my front teeth missing as a result of a fight I'd had leading up to my detention. In the words of another one of my friend's poems:

And the muscles of his body tighten. His temper rises and
a force from somewhere that he will never understand
gives him his mighty strength.

In those days, when I looked into the mirror I was greeted by a good-looking man with piercing blue eyes, just like my father's. These days I am greeted with a reflection that has endured many seasons with too many late nights – and although my once black hair is slowly but gently greying, my face thankfully hasn't given up on smiling. My inner torment was buried within my soul, far too deep to reach and deeper still to understand, but I doubt if anyone missed the scars on both my wrists, that captured the outward signs of my angst at the time.

I just kept plodding along in life and I can only hope that I have reached a point where I have made sense of my abusive childhood by having disengaged from the destructive influences that blighted my earlier life. Not as many people are hospitalised these days as they were in the past. Care in the Community has meant that out-patient clinics have become the norm in Ireland. But even in these clinics you can see real emotional suffering. It is ever-present on people's faces and in their eyes. I have formed a silent allegiance with many fellow patients because I know they are in a similar situation to me. I also get the opportunity to listen to people's experiences and occasionally make friends. One such friend, like me, has had bipolar since her late teens but unlike me, who has only self-harmed to release my stresses, has tried to commit suicide many times. Like me, she too has looked for acceptance all her life by continuously searching for someone to love, but unlike me she settled for a partner who she does not love. She once confided in me that the pain of her past prevents her from consummating the marriage. Her husband has become a father figure but he in return is content, respecting her wishes.

I have learned to keep my visions and perceptions to myself. Quite the contrary to being a burden, they often bring reassurance and comfort. I know I am not insane when I see dead people. I was about eight when I first started seeing them. I remember waking up one night and seeing the image of a tall, thin figure standing at the foot of my bed, but not feeling the least bit afraid. It seemed normal right from the beginning. Of course, others didn't agree and when I told members of my family I was mocked, told to 'shut up', accused of telling fairytales or in the words of my mother, it was just a nightmare that seemed real. I rarely tell others now because although their words may seem to indicate that they understand, their tone is usually patronising and besides their faces always tell me how freaked out they feel.

I also know that it is highly unlikely that I have bipolar disorder. I stopped drinking ten years ago, yet the diagnosis is still hung around my neck like a gold medallion. I rarely take the medication and usually burn them in the kitchen range. I pretend I take them to pacify my psychiatrist because I claim disability allowance, which requires renewal forms to be completed. Please don't think badly of me. I don't claim this money through dishonesty or because I'm lazy. I need to live and without it I would live in poverty. Nobody wants to employ me as I am viewed as soiled goods. I am a man with a past who has done bad things and said bad things. I have badly beaten people, insulted them and behaved in some very undignified ways during my drinking years that have left scars, not just on my arms, but on my character, and on my soul. But what I have also learned in the last few years is that you can be alone and be neither happy nor unhappy – but content, which is a form of happiness in itself. I don't think of the future. I think of the present. What will come, will come by itself. Every minute, everyday can be a new beginning if you want it to be. In the words of Buddha, from whose writings I have gained much inspiration, 'No matter how hard the past, you can always begin again.'

Life with bipolar is not a bowl of cherries, but:

1. I have a strong faith in God
2. I accept my illness
3. I take care of my mental and spiritual welfare
4. I keep active and busy
5. I'm becoming aware of stress (learning to say 'No')
6. I am able to talk about my illness
7. I never feel ashamed of it
8. I have the ability to laugh at my life
9. I feel blessed to being well today
10. I am in control and at peace.

Stephanie

Jennifer

If I were to write a letter to my parents, I would word it something like this:

> *Thank you for the wonderful childhood. It was bloody great. I enjoyed every single moment being in all those care homes. I remember my eleventh birthday, alone and wondering what I had done wrong not to receive a card or present from you. Yes, thank you so very much indeed.*

It's not that I have any inclination to write to either of them. My mother has lived in Australia for the past ten years. There have been no letters or telephone calls, not even a Christmas card. I see my father's face a little too often, not helped by the fact that he only lives two miles away. He writes me letters all the time.

"The Mental Health Team will section you, unless you take your medication," he wrote in his last letter.

And the one before that: "Your tablets are to prevent you from saying horribly untruthful things."

I like Jacinta, my social worker. The three words that I would use to describe her would be: tall, blonde and elegant. Bit of a cliché really. I'd never tell her that though, because we have a love-hate relationship. She has a very sharp wit and speaks in a posh voice. I always wonder what she is going to be wearing before I meet her: will it be slacks or skirt, high heels or boots, plunging neckline or roll-up sweater. But it is her posh accent that lingers most in my mind. I constantly imitate her voice at home. "Oh Jennifer, you must get a grip," I say to the bathroom mirror, all the time. "You must drink more water – have you eaten? Oh you must eat." When I was in the supermarket the other day, I even thanked the check-out boy in my best Jacinta impersonation. "Oh thank you *soooooo* much, you're awfully kind, but you must get a grip," as he handed me back my change. The poor boy was shocked and stared at me in total bewilderment.

Jacinta liked my new thong. "Purple suits you," she said.

I love wearing tutus. It was one of my sisters who introduced me to them one day when I was at her flat and I accidentally spilt coffee down my jeans. I loved the freedom and the feeling of liberation I felt when I first put one on and from that day forward there was no turning back. Jacinta agrees with me that wearing one is far more stylish than wearing a tracksuit. But there are nasty people who wouldn't agree with this. I hate going on buses because I am guaranteed to get hassle from people.

"Not quite a ballerina yet?" one person said to me, to which another idiot mouthed, "Sorry love, but is there something wrong with your wiring?"

One day, I saw an ambulance passing my house. It was going at such speed that I panicked and thought my sister had been in an accident. I ran out of the house and jogged to Jacinta's office, which is four miles away. She was both annoyed and full of questions.

"Why do you think it might be your sister? You'll give yourself a heart attack with all this running, you must get a grip – you must ring her? Here, use my phone to call her now." I discovered it wasn't my sister in the ambulance after all. Phew, I let out a great sigh of relief.

Jacinta isn't always nice though. In fact, she can be bitchy and spiteful at times. I had been painting my kitchen when I accidentally dropped my hammer into the paint can. It happened all of a flash. One second I was painting the wall over the cooker a deep red colour when I reached over for the hammer to remove a nail from the wall. I dropped the bloody hammer and it fell into the paint. I nearly screamed with terror. I quickly picked it out of the can, only to realise that the hammer was completely covered in paint. I wasn't drunk. Okay, I'd had a few vodkas to give me Dutch courage before I started the painting. Before I knew it, the whole thing had turned into chaos. I couldn't find my flip-flops and so had to run barefoot to Jacinta's office to show her the hammer, which looked like it was covered in blood. It was around Halloween time and I thought she would see the funny side of my antic.

The interrogation began the moment I walked through the door.

"Are you feeling unwell?"

"You have lost *soooooo* much weight. Why are you drinking lemon juice?" she said.

"Have you any idea what Olazapine does to you?" I replied before adding, "No, I thought not."

I knew she wouldn't care if I was twenty stone as long as she had her slim figure.

"But you'll be skeletal if you carry on like this," she replied.

"Then you'll have to accompany me to Anorexics Anonymous, won't you?" I replied. "We can sit there and share our stories in our best voices, it will be *soooooo* cool."

My quip was not met with a smile but I didn't care because I wasn't going to let her get away with her snide attitude. But Jacinta doesn't like to be outwitted and later that afternoon I received my punishment when she turned up at my flat with a psychiatrist, a ginger bearded man who introduced himself as Frederick. I burst out giggling when I heard his name. He frowned in return. My father came along with them too, but when I saw him I started screaming. I didn't know and can't even remember what I was saying. It felt like I had no control of the words, as if someone was inside my head pushing them out and all I had to do was oblige by opening my mouth.

"Don't let him near me!" were my last words before I was walked to the ambulance.

My father dominated my last review meeting, interrupting people as they spoke and telling everyone what a difficult child I had been. I couldn't have been that difficult, but it made me wonder afterwards if I could discover what I was really like by asking Jacinta to get permission for me to read my medical notes. I was given my file to read, but much of what it included made little sense. Besides, its contents only contained information after my eighteenth birthday. I wanted to read about my childhood. I was hoping I would find out why I had such a poor relationship with my father – and why he thought I was bad. I kept thinking that maybe I would discover that maybe I did something horrible when I was a child and that was the reason why he always saw me in a bad light.

My first visitor to the hospital was the elegant traitor, otherwise known as Jacinta.

"You look *soooooo* much better," she said.

I didn't reply because I sometimes think I shouldn't trust her as much as I do, that she is on my father's side – his mole.

"We all know you self-medicate with vodka. Why not take your real medication for three weeks, stop for three weeks, then take them for another three before stopping again and so on and so forth. As long as you have a steady stream of medication in your body, you won't relapse," she said.

"Thank you Doctor Jacinta!" I replied.

Guess what? I met a man in hospital who I liked and he, wait for this, became my boyfriend. Charlie was cool, a great kisser but he turned out to be a bit strange. One day we were out walking in town while on day release when he saw two men standing outside a pub who he instantly thought were talking about us. He insisted on going up and challenging them. I felt so embarrassed by his aggressiveness, and then afterwards he turned on me and told me he felt aggrieved when I didn't support him. He then shouted out to everyone in the street that he no longer wanted to be my boyfriend, leaving me wondering what I had done wrong.

I'm now single again, but out of hospital. Jacinta is encouraging me to do some voluntary work. It is only a couple of days doing some conservation work and gardening. Some days I help tidy the local cemetery or plant trees and sow flowers in the park.

Jacinta thinks I should apply for a job in ecology because I am passionate about recycling and hate the way people cause so much waste in their environment. It is good that we are on amicable terms again.

"I want to contribute to society and not be a scrounger," I told her.

"You have such great potential," she replied.

I'm resting at home today. The radio is on in the background. I'm listening to Classic FM which is playing *Eroica*, which happens to be my favourite of Beethoven's symphonies. I feel calm as I take sips of my cranberry and elderflower tea. The world of mania feels calm. It feels like the world is taking a deep breath and is relaxed. On the table next to me is an unopened letter from my father which arrived this morning. I'm contemplating not opening it. Ideally, I would like to tear it into a million tiny pieces but curiosity is lurking at the back of my mind, wondering what he has to say this time. But why should I care? I know he only wants to upset me because that is what bastards do – they upset people. But for now I will resist temptation and leave it there to stew for at least a little while longer.

Brian

Carers worry about the future and think they are selfish when they wonder if they will be the only one taking care of their loved one in years to come. They feel fear because they don't know what the next day will bring because of the volatility of the illness. They feel used because someone with bipolar who wants to get his/her own way can use the condition for this purpose. There is guilt at feeling inadequate for not doing more to help them get well. Anger, too, plays a part, especially in families where there is no support forthcoming from other family members, because they feel embarrassed. Then there is the mental exhaustion from both the physical care and the emotional strain of worrying that they will harm themselves. Fears exist in families, wondering if it is genetic and if children in the family will go on to develop bipolar in adulthood. But most of all there is love. Deep love, despite everything else. This has to be present, because looking after someone with bipolar is emotionally strenuous.

The city beckoned after we were married in 1968, when I was twenty-three and Margaret was nineteen, and we have lived here ever since. Her parents thought we were too young to get married, but we were childhood sweethearts since school. I knew from the moment when I first started noticing girls that Margaret was the one for me. But after we had been married for two years, there were signs that something was wrong. Margaret worked long hours as a civil servant and generally liked her job, but one winter in the early seventies a flu epidemic spread rapidly, and only those with the strongest immune systems seemed to evade its grasp. Margaret was sick for weeks. On top of that we were about to move into our newly purchased first home, which made matters very stressful. In hindsight, there were tell-tale signs before this, but I paid little attention to them – partly because I had never encountered anything like this before, but mainly because Margaret never complained of feeling depressed. I was a mechanic and used to work half-days on Saturday. When I came home in the early afternoon, Margaret would still be in bed. I thought she was just tired and having a lie-in because it was the weekend, but looking back I can see it was more than that, because after she'd get up, she wouldn't have any interest or incentive to do anything for the remainder of the day. She went to the doctor and he gave her some tablets. A few weeks later she took an overdose and nearly succeeded in dying.

Margaret was taken to a psychiatric hospital located in a rural location. It had a farm attached where patients helped out in the vegetable gardens or cleaning out chicken pens and feeding straw to the horses as part of their recovery process. I got a telephone call from the hospital asking me to come in and speak to the psychiatrist. He told me she was suffering from *Manic Depression,* but said this would be treated with a special kind of medication. I was young, naïve and walked away feeling relieved, happy she was going to be cured and afterwards would come home and things would go back to normal. How wrong was I? The past forty years have taken on the same pattern. Every time she puts one foot forward, she takes two steps backwards. We have seen highs followed by lows, lows followed by highs and a combination of both – blips during which she managed to escape hospitalisation by the skin of her teeth but overall, there have been very few periods when she has reached a point where she could be considered well. Welcome to the world of Brian and Margaret and please accept my invitation as I take you through her journey of an illness that has seen dozens of psychiatrists treat her with dozens of medications, believing they would heal her emotional distress, as well as fifty electroconvulsive therapy treatments in an attempt to lift her out of deep depressions. All of this could be forgiven and forgotten if Margaret was now cured. Admittedly, at times, medication has either calmed her mania down or raised her moods a little – but she now presents as a sad and lonely figure with a constant apathetic look on her face – as well as being confined to a wheelchair and requiring twenty-four hour care.

Margaret mainly suffers from two types of mania – or at least this is how it appears from my viewpoint. Sometimes she lives life as if she were on a cloud or another planet. In the days that precede a manic phase, her skin glows more healthily; her posture allows her to sit upright in the wheelchair as if her shoulders have been removed from shackles. Her voice even seems to take on a more confident pitch, giving her a happy, gregarious and carefree attitude. She obsessively orders goods from catalogues and spends money like a teenager who knows little of its value. She spends on clothes, household items, and china trinkets of every description. Once she sees something she likes, she buys it. Needless to say our house is brimming to the rafters with unwanted goods that are neither used nor needed. The other type of mania is her angry phase, in which she turns against people, including myself, neighbours and any visitor to our home. Her paranoia becomes so intense that she thinks people are either plotting, criticising or laughing at her behind her back, but to try and convince her otherwise only leads to confrontation. The yelling and swearing can continue for hours, so I have found staying silent is the best way of dealing with this.

As previously mentioned, the past forty years have seen a lot of medications prescribed one minute and stopped the next and, like the psychiatrists who have come and gone, they have formed a distinct pattern that never seems to vary. Each new tablet and each different psychiatrist brings a glimmer of hope until the moment of realisation arrives and you know neither has made any difference. Indeed, if all the medication she has been prescribed over the years was counted out, there would enough to open up a pharmacy, but none of it has worked – or is likely to work. Advice and encouragement given by each psychiatrist is like a ship sailing through the night, because when Margaret returns for a check-up, the psychiatrist she saw the last time will have gone and a stranger will be sitting in their place making yet more changes, more suggestions and justifying changes of medications or the necessity to experiment in order to best stabilise the condition. But nothing seems to stabilise her.

She has been on and off Lithium numerous times. It is her current medication, despite giving her constant tremors and a massive appetite. The other mainstays were a regime of Depakote and Haloperidol, which led to her having seizures and falls, resulting in neurological tests showing brain damage which manifested itself in the disorientation that will always now remain, hence her becoming wheelchair-bound.

My health took a dip last year from the sheer exhaustion of looking after her for many years. I wasn't sleeping at night, but being a proud man I didn't want to appear needy and reach out for help. I thought I could manage all by myself, but I collapsed and was taken to hospital, where at first it was thought I'd had a stroke. Thankfully, I hadn't and I've completely recovered. This crisis brought about an unexpected bonus though, resulting in Adult Social Services assigning a care package consisting of round-the-clock care for Margaret. In some ways, I had to concede defeat by not being able to look after her by myself any longer, but I look back with pride over the years of love that bonded us together, which undoubtedly gave me the strength to stay when other men may have found themselves without enough love or capability.

The carers do a good job of looking after Margaret but I still do the shopping and prepare our evening meal. We relax after supper with me usually falling asleep reading the newspaper, while some music plays softly in the background. We take every day as it comes. That's our fate. We can never plan for the future – one day at a time – but we are thankful that things are ticking along as well as they are. Let me assure anyone not already convinced though that living with someone with bipolar is not a nice life. I do sometimes sit and wonder about the journey life bestowed on Margaret. If a new doctor walked into our house today and said he would be able to cure Margaret of bipolar, I would laugh out loud and say, "I'll believe that when I see it." But on the other hand, I have no option but to trust the medical profession, although it is clear the mysteriousness of the condition has beaten them in finding an answer, as much as it has beaten the will of ordinary people like Margaret in ever hoping that their lives will be free of it.

Words in a text message that best describe my bipolar:

1. Exhilarating
2. Petrifying
3. Revealing
4. Unpredictable
5. Despair
6. Uninvited
7. Entrapment
8. Apathy
9. Powerless
10. Alone.

Dylan

Lucy

I'm just finishing my degree in Fine Art and specialise in sculpture. I've enjoyed the challenge of working together with other professionals in putting together an exhibition showcasing some of my proudest creations. I smile and am cheerful to the outside world, and those who don't know me think I'm someone who is happy and carefree. Only a few select friends know about my bipolar. As for others, why should they know my business?

I was only fourteen but I knew something was wrong. I was moody and had few friends, resulting in me mainly spending time alone in my bedroom, staring into space. I was convinced there was something strange about me but the GP said I was too young to be prescribed antidepressants. I staggered on through that maze throughout my final school years and into early adulthood. I went to Jersey when I was twenty-one – and put all my effort and energy into my administration job. I craved acceptance and wanted to be liked by everyone in the office. The word no was void in my vocabulary because I feared disappointing people. I was still a virgin and wanted to explore and learn more about life and myself. I embraced nightclubs with a passion and slept with several men. I learned to live and to have fun and was thrilled at the enjoyment that life unwrapped for me. I was first introduced to cannabis and ecstasy around that time and believed I benefited from them with my newly acquired confidence. In reality, they only helped mask my difficulties, because stress in my job started to build up and eventually took such a hold that I crumbed under its weight. I swiftly returned home and shortly afterwards had my first breakdown.

I started to self-harm by scratching my wrists. This initially brought relief from the feeling of being trapped in my own mind, but it was not enough to sustain me. One day, the despair became so great that I reached for some painkillers and took them with some of my father's poitín*. I didn't want to live, but on the other hand I didn't want to die. It felt like I was being pulled down by a heavy weight tied around my waist. My mind began to feel programmed, like someone who was living in a parallel universe. I had become an onlooker who just sat around at home and gazed at life, thinking it was outside of my control to take part in it. My parents became so worried they had me hospitalised. There I was kept under lock and key twenty-four hours a day. Hospital was a wretched place, confusing, frightening and full of misery – like entering a dark cave with only a small flashlight for guidance, coupled with the foreboding feeling that you were lost, abandoned – never to be found again.

After discharge, my community psychiatric nurse placed me on a day release programme – where I was made to associate with people with all kinds of mental health problems, as well as drug addicts. When I protested against it, I was bluntly told that the root of all mental problems was the same and that I was no different to anyone else in the group. But I knew this to be untrue and failed to identify with some of their illnesses and addictions, so I stopped attending. I knew what was wrong and that the answer to my problems would never come from that group. I was depressed, full of feelings of not being good enough – bright enough – happy enough – successful enough. I wasn't craving drugs. I just had bad feelings about my life, coupled with parents who didn't understand. Don't get me wrong – they are lovely people, but their values are different to mine. I have always believed in education but to them getting a job, saving money, getting married and having children are the only things in life that matter.

There was a seven-year gap in between my first breakdown and my second, which occurred when I became elated in Australia. I had taken antidepressants on and off over the years but escaped Lithium and other antipsychotic and mood stabilising medications. However, they lay in waiting for me, but not before I completed my return trip with my partner. It started with the feeling that everything was great and everyone was fabulous. I was full of 'Down Under' euphoria for its glorious sunshine and unlimited beaches. I was always on the go – working long hours – but was always distracted by events going on around me. I drank champagne as I lay on the beach and occasionally smoked cannabis in the belief that it would calm me when the strain of work spilt over into my relationship, causing arguments, but it failed to do this. Things got worse and I split up from my partner but we decided to remain friends. However, we both missed home, not helped by our break-up and my increasing mania, prompting us to return home earlier than planned. I slipped back into depression and over a period of a couple of months getting upset and being tearful the whole time came to feel normal. I also became plagued with fears about the future and whether I would ever meet someone and be able to fall in love again. Anxieties refused to budge, and then I did what I had done seven years earlier and reached for the painkillers and bottle of poitín, which resulted in a second hospitalisation. One of the good things to come out of this though, was that my partner visited me, enabling us to talk and sort out our differences. We decided to give our relationship another go and have been together now for thirteen years.

Although it was good to be reconciled with my partner, I was apprehensive about leaving the safety of the hospital and returning home, fearing that I'd become unwell again. I hated the idea. There is a distinct lack of resources for people coming out of hospital in my home town but I was extremely fortunate that my local hospital placed me on a recovery programme that helped me focus on my recovery and make future plans. I enrolled on a FETAC* life-skills training course, which I attended for a year and a half. The course taught people to set attainable goals against their strengths. It even went one step further by pushing people to think outside their comfort zones in order to develop new ideas and opportunities. The FETAC course had many plus points in the sense that it re-introduced normality into my life and allowed me to plan my future in a way that I had never contemplated before. I saw a psychologist around the same time who firmly prompted me to take the leap from procrastination to action. The next day I telephoned around various colleges asking for prospectuses. A couple of months later I started my degree and the journey to achieving my biggest ever achievement.

I still detest Lithium, because for years it made me feel so nauseous every night and I blamed it for my underactive thyroid, that makes me feel tired much of the time. Psychiatrists come and go in my local hospital because of funding, although the current one seems to have stayed longer than her predecessors, which is a shame because I believe she is so removed from life and people, to the degree you could walk into her clinic with one of your limbs falling off, and she wouldn't bat an eyelid. When I complained to her about how I was feeling, I interpreted her stare as, "What do you expect me to do about that?" She followed this with a verbal rebuke: "Isn't it better that you are well." I got around this problem eventually by drinking lots of water: the more hydrated I am the easier it is for my system to tolerate the Lithium. I feel I will be on medication for the rest of my life. In one sense this fills me with dread – but then I think that at least I am living with a managed disease that won't kill me by itself.

Bipolar is an unusual illness in the sense that it can have many admirers or none at all. It can make you loud and bashful or quiet and retiring. It always invites itself into your circle and becomes a visitor who overstays its welcome. Love or loathe it – and I have felt both – it is part of me that I have accepted, painfully, reluctantly yet peacefully. It wears a coat of many colours but I am happy and grateful that my wardrobe of emotion has dressed itself in the best garment of all – tolerance. And it is with this that I now live my life.

Poitín is a highly alcoholic beverage (60–95% abv), which is distilled from malted barley, grain or potatoes. It is one of the strongest alcoholic drinks in the world and is still illegal in some countries.

FETAC – Further Education and Training Awards Council is the statutory awarding body for further education in Ireland. FETAC was established on 11th June 2001 under the Qualifications (Education and Training) Act 1999.

Jarlath

In my opinion, being both bipolar and gay is not a good combination, because they cause stress in different ways and sometimes at the same time. I came out to my parents and siblings fifteen years ago. Although there was a slight change I guess in the way we saw and spoke to each other, their reactions were mainly positive. The idea of what it is to be gay comes with preconceived ideas of not conforming to the norms of society. Furthermore, there is the dreaded fear in Ireland of homosexuality, following clerical child abuse that has unfortunately sometimes led homosexuality to be confused with paedophilia. Coming out should have been a huge relief because I had this burden hanging over me all during my teenage years. I never wanted to grow up because I thought getting older would mean being exposed to realities that I wanted to avoid. I was a quiet teenager – always on guard and avoiding plans for the future, fearing failure and disappointment. The result of this was that life was going ahead without me – aimlessly heading towards a chasm of its own. But it should have been going somewhere dynamic, where I would've been happy. This much I knew despite my continuous analysis of situations; but my mind failed to deal with the pressure and instead it unravelled. Then, three weeks after telling everyone I was gay and just shortly after my twenty-second birthday, I became so manic and paranoid, believing everyone was making fun of me behind my back, that I spent the next four months in hospital.

Some of the male nurses were really cute. I felt so lucky to be surrounded by their gorgeous presence that it made up for being locked away in hospital. There was one nurse in particular who stood out with his well-toned six-pack. Indeed, his abdominal features preoccupied my thoughts and my depression felt lighter on days when he was working. It almost felt a drudge leaving him behind after I was discharged. I faced life again with the help of a psychologist who talked me through what it was like to be gay. As I said, coming out wasn't the big release that I had expected it to be. I was just as lonely as beforehand, but my counsellor helped me overcome my social awkwardness and on one occasion took me to a gay bar to get me used to living a gay lifestyle. The atmosphere felt unthreatening. I embraced its safety and began to make friends and feel happier, more content and accepting of my sexuality, when something unimaginable happened. I gradually started getting fewer and fewer erections and then they completely stopped. The antidepressants caused my impotence. I didn't know what to do and felt resentment at having the need to take the medication that caused my newfound disability and sudden lack of interest in sex. I took a step back from the gay scene and began to isolate myself from friends because I was too embarrassed to tell them the truth. Telling them about my medication would reveal my bipolar – which I didn't want to risk. Instead, I tolerated accusations of being too precious and feeling better than others when I turned down offers for sex. I struggled on like this for three years ago, but I was very fortunate to then meet my partner, who understands my situation and illness.

I found true love in my new boyfriend and felt like life had started all over again, only this time it was better. It helped that I pushed myself to change and overcame the negative thoughts I held about myself. I returned to college in my early thirties to study economics, which is a move I am so pleased I took, because the feeling of accomplishment compensates for the hospital admissions, Lithium and antidepressants. Before becoming a mature student, I had managed to hold a few jobs down – but the greatest shortfall in these was the lack of understanding about mental health in the workplace. It is still considered taboo to take time off to deal with depression. There's no problem when a person telephones work sick with a cold or stomach bug – or has a period off for planned surgery. But the moment any mental issue comes to the surface, it is not accepted in the same vein. The depressive side of my bipolar comes and goes and I have no control over it. Sometimes it lasts a few days – sometimes weeks but never longer than two months. Depression is a challenging illness that needs time and patience because, when it's mixed with stress, it exacerbates the problem even further, making recovery longer.

My family have become less supportive as I've grown older – and if I'm frank, have probably been more supportive about me being gay than they have been with my bipolar. I accept that my parents are getting older and have started to lessen their grip on me now that I have settled down with my partner. But the last few years has seen my parents and my siblings distance themselves from me when I become unwell. I am lucky if I get a "How are you?" because they fear me opening up about my feelings. My brothers and sisters are all married with children and are wrapped up in their own lives and worries – and removing them from their bubble makes them feel uncomfortable. It's like giving an over-worked stressed employee more tasks to do. The collapse of the economy made people less compassionate towards others because everyone was suddenly consumed with debts. This was hard to accept at first – but now I have accepted this as part of life, knowing that it is a myth to think any family is perfect.

Ireland has its fair share of empty sentiment. Admittedly, there is less shame on the one hand for people speaking out about their mental health problems in public, but the media for some reason puts a happy slant on this. I continuously see people on television speaking about their illness in the past tense, in a way that suggests they have beaten some adversity like drug addiction or alcoholism. Take depression, for example. I recently saw someone speaking about how well they were currently feeling, which was a good thing to hear, but what they didn't say was how they cope on days when they feel miserable and haven't any inclination to face the world. The media doesn't tell you that bipolar comes and goes. It doesn't tell you that inbetween episodes of mania and depression, people take lengthy periods to recover. Of course you need to acknowledge periods of good health because, like episodes of illness, these will be times when a person can function normally, albeit within the remits of what the side-effects and fears of becoming unwell again dictate.

Visits to my psychiatrist are like visits to the bank manager. It is a business arrangement, because he bears all the hallmarks of a meticulous businessman who is careful of everything he says, fearing he will be accused of saying or doing something wrong. It is like getting a refusal for an extension to an overdraft, as he doesn't agree with any of my viewpoints on reducing, changing or abandoning the antidepressants I am taking – although I have been frank with him about my erectile dysfunction and the fear I have of losing my partner because of this. I asked him to recommend a counsellor for me so that I can have more counselling but instead of recommending someone he knew, he just printed off a list of names from the internet – which I could have easily done myself at home. So here I am in limbo. Most people take things, including their lives and their future, for granted – but living with bipolar does not allow this luxury. You have to make a special effort to face it – to force yourself to feel *normal*, to cast aside its frustrations and hope you survive the cliff hangers and trials it throws at you, so that you can live another day and be able to tell your story.

10 Sentences that describe my bipolar life:

1. Living with bipolar disorder can be like living your life to the absolute fullest, coupled with not living at all.

2. It can be the best illness in the world and the most limiting illness in your life.

3. It's impossible to utilise the positives of this illness without enduring the negatives.

4. Medication stifles the positive attributes that I would love to keep, especially the excessive energy, enthusiasm and new unique ideas, and leaves you feeling zombified and lazy!

5. The aftermath or a manic episode makes it impossible to refuse medication.

6. You end up taking medication just to keep everyone else happy.

7. The temptation to come off my meds will always be there.

8. To avoid future episodes I have had to make changes to my lifestyle as well as being consistent with my antipsychotics.

9. I am constantly aware and paranoid about what others think of me.

10. I will always be aware when undertaking any new venture that I am deemed unreliable, due to the nature of this illness.

Virginia

Maire

My best friend is my youngest daughter, Claire, who has Down's Syndrome. We laugh so much together, sometimes at the silliest little things and we both love going to shows. I've lost count of the number of times we've seen *Grease* and *Blood Brothers* and just like Claire, I never tire of their stories. She was placed in foster care for several years when my bipolar first took hold. My eldest daughter, Veronica, went to live with her father, from whom I had separated and with whom I was barely on speaking terms. After my health stabilised, Claire returned to live with me, while Veronica remained living with her father and over time grew closer to him. The opposite happened to she and I, to the extent that a detachment exists between us to this very day. Maybe her father turned her against me, but I never argued with him and we managed to be civil to each other whenever he and Veronica came to visit Claire – but in the years leading up to his death, he barely featured in my life apart from these infrequent visits. He died of cirrhosis after a long battle with the disease. I didn't go to his funeral, nor did I feel sad or guilty at his death because I believed at that stage we did not owe each other anything. He was ten years older, which was part of the attraction. My father died when I was young, making me yearn for a father figure – someone strong and caring, someone who would take care of me. I knew no better. But instead of him caring for me I carried him. I worked nights at a nursing home, often finding myself coming home after long shifts and having to stay awake to comfort him through the delirium tremens which made him shake uncontrollably after a night of heavy drinking. He thought I had grown oblivious to the sight of lipstick on cigarette ends in the ashtray and to unexplained stains on the sheets. He was devious. I didn't nickname him 'The Fox' for nothing – but somehow his cheating managed to stretch my sanity to the point where I became bulimic and although I still stayed with him and Veronica and Claire, we never married. Looking back now, I can see we were two sick people who weren't good for each other and while we had some happy times on family picnics during sober periods, I knew deep down his womanising meant he'd never be able to commit to anyone.

I wrote to Veronica after the funeral, telling her that I loved her and said I hoped she didn't feel I preferred or loved Claire more than her. She never replied but I received an invitation to her wedding the following year. I attended, but felt like a stranger. Her father's name was mentioned in the wedding service, and afterwards at the reception during the speeches, but there was no mention of me, leaving me wondering if I had been airbrushed out of the story. But there is something about my relationship with Veronica that reminds me of the one I have with my own mother. Even though my mother is now an old woman now living in a care home, it is a big effort for me to pick up the phone to ring her, because I feel no love towards her. An older neighbour abused me as a child but she always refused to believe me, making me cast my dark little secret into a box and place it on a shelf in the back of my head. There it remained hidden but not forgotten, because you never forget where you store something like that.

My bipolar first surfaced in the early nineties with high bursts of energy that I attributed to stress working in a busy city centre train station. Suddenly one day it was as if a spring cracked open in my head. It started with idiotic antics, like putting a five pound note on a plate and exclaiming out loud, "I've got money to burn," before setting fire to it. I became obsessed with white cars and had to see two of them, as with magpies, before considering them to be a sign of good luck. One day I went up to the loft, unwrapped my old communion dress and asked Veronica, who was ten at the time, to change into it. I believed that the world was soon coming to an end and wanted to show people how angelic she was before the final damnation – parading her up and down the street for everyone to see. No-one could convince me that the world wasn't going to end, making me think it was extra sensory perception that enabled only me to anticipate the second coming of Jesus. I thought people needed God in their lives and started delivering medals, holy pictures and prayer leaflets to every house in my neighbourhood and beyond. At home, I started clearing everything out of the house because I couldn't see the point of having possessions when paradise was looming. I walked around town, handing out lumps of sugar to people who appeared unhappy in the hope of making them sweeter, nicer people before they entered the kingdom of God. I still joke with my best friend about this when I see someone who appears miserable, often saying something like, "That one definitely needs a little sugar," which we laugh about as I recount the madness, the sheer lunacy of my reasoning at that time.

These days, while I no longer have full-blown manic episodes, I nonetheless live with a relative degree of mania and manage this by keeping myself busy, although I sometimes get fearful that any stress will make me become unwell again. Even when it swaps over to depression, I am not a person who lies in bed for lengthy periods. I do voluntary work three days a week with Oxfam and enjoy serving in the shop and talking to people. I make necklaces and earrings and sell these in the shop and donate the proceeds. A friend introduced me to aromatherapy sessions, which I go to every fortnight, and have discovered that scents like frankincense, lavender and rose help me relax. But it is my community psychiatric nurse who has been my saviour, helping me put my childhood sexual abuse into perspective. Through her support and counselling I have been able to open the box stored deep at the back of my mind and examine its contents – without fear or bitterness – but with a realisation that it is not only the perpetrator who can never inflict hurt on me again, it is every other person too.

I have loads of friends, young and old, mainly because there is a strong sense of community in my neighbourhood. Going to daily Mass is a big part of my routine as my faith has sustained me during times when I felt the darkness over my horizon would never lift. In the past I became overweight but have discovered exercise and sensible eating helps keep obesity at bay. My current medication is Lithium and Haloperidol, which I began taking after my last breakdown five years ago. I suspect one of the side-effects of these is memory loss because there has been at least a twenty per cent deterioration in my memory over the past couple of years, but ultimately it is difficult to determine when and what caused this because since my bipolar started I have spent many periods in hospital combating the highs and the lows – and the lows and the highs – and every time I was hospitalised I became the guinea pig for a new tablet to see if it would help. I have reached a point where my moods seem to have evened out. To be well is to be in control – and to be unwell is the opposite. But bipolar has a mind of its own. It is a condition of extremes, a feast or a famine, war or peace; but mainly moments range from noisy activity to deadly silence. There is only a certain amount a person can do to prevent a relapse. I strive to achieve this and if ever I need reassurance of how well I'm doing, I take a look at Claire and realise how grateful I am for the happiness we share together.

William

I was a twenty-seven year old college lecturer when in 1964 I first experienced depression. I went to my GP and asked him if I could see a psychiatrist.

"The trouble with you is that you've been watching too many television programmes," he replied.

I know this now sounds ludicrous, but requests like this were unusual in the 1960s. He gave me a prescription for amphetamines and explained these would soon make me feel better. Unfortunately, the drugs failed to help and left me feeling terrible, with a continuous dry mouth, constipation and tremors. Afterwards, I went to psychotherapy and group therapy before finally becoming a disciple of Osho – who was an Indian spiritual guru (1931–1990) who drew followers in large numbers from all over the world to his Ashram in Pune. There, they were put into groups to meditate in order to seek the answer to the only question that Osho said matters – "Who am I?"

Over the next decade I travelled with Osho to his communes in India, Japan, New Zealand and Amsterdam. Deep down I was convinced that if I found the right way to live, I would cease to be depressed. Even during the worst times I clung onto the hope that one day I would be free of this nightmare. My ambition became a relentless quest to find the answer to that all-important question of who I was, rendering me in total awe of Osho's wisdom, mysticism and serenity, but he rebuked me and others in the commune when he said, "Don't look at my finger, look at the moon," and "Don't watch me, watch the wonderful image in the sky." At first I failed to understand the meaning of these statements, but over time realised how important it is to be present in the moment by not being buried in the past or digging too deep into the future. I learned through him that we take on other peoples' definitions of ourselves. We have to move away from our parents, friends and society to discover, without distraction, the deeper meaning of ourselves. My time with Osho left me with fewer doubts about myself. I saw glimpses of the real me and developed a deeper understanding of what it entails to be a survivor. That doesn't mean that I no longer have moments of panic or worry, but rather reflects a feeling of knowing that I will overcome difficulties without succumbing to them.

My last manic episode occurred in my daughter's house eleven years ago. She, her brother, friends and I were eating dinner when I started telling them the 'Truths' of life in an unstoppable rant. Nothing deflected me from dominating the conversation. My daughter's best friend, a young gay male, asked me a question which I interpreted as a snide put-down, resulting in me swearing at him and calling him a queer. There was a pained silence. My daughter told me the next day how disgusted she was at my behaviour. That was the wake-up call that I needed because, rather amazingly, as the days went by I saw clearly for the first time in my life that I was manic. It's become difficult to imagine how I thought the high moods I had previously experienced were normal, particularly as they had ranged from physical threats to colleagues to periods of seemingly inexhaustible energy.

After the incident at my daughter's house I turned to my consultant for help. Osho has often used the words, "Real change only occurs during a crisis," and how correct he was. I was riddled with guilt and ashamed of my verbal attack on my daughter's friend. I was placed on Lithium, which helped calm me down. However, one of the unfortunate side-effects was weight gain. Within two years I ballooned out to over 18 stone. But after taking Lithium for five years, I was convinced I had made a full recovery. I felt so good that it seemed natural to immediately stop taking it. I ignored literature advising against this because such action guarantees a major relapse within six months. This indeed became a reality because within weeks I was manic again – ranting, argumentative and driven by conflict and excitability. My psychiatrist put me back on Lithium and within a fortnight I made a dramatic recovery.

Leaving bipolar aside for the moment, my main irritant of recent years has been the antisocial neighbours who moved into the flat above me. I tried to be reasonable and to settle my grievance with them amicably but their shouting, screaming, drinking and sex sounds were relentless. They wouldn't accept they were doing anything wrong and often shouted in my letterbox that I was an interfering old git. I reported the matter to the police. They did nothing. I went to the Council. They were equally useless with their superficial, "We'll sort it out," but nothing ever came of their promise. A nasty acquaintance, who knew of my mental condition, heard what was going on and reported me to my psychiatrist, claiming that I was becoming unwell. I was summoned to a terse meeting. Instantly, it felt like he had made up his mind about the state of my health beforehand. He never asked me how I'd been since our last meeting with him. If so, I would have told him that I had been waking up depressed for over a week with the stress and noise of the neighbours. Instead, he chose to tell me I was manic because I was expressing anger about the stress I was under. I refuted his analysis, which made him frown. I would have appreciated a little credibility, an acknowledgment that I knew my illness well enough not to confuse ordinary anger with a manic episode. I asked him to explain his definition of anger, but he didn't answer. Shortly afterwards, I received good news. My complaint, which was referred to the ombudsman, found in my favour that my rights had been violated and berated the Council's failure to deal with the antisocial behaviour. The Police Complaints Commission also upheld a complaint about the failure of the police to deal with an incident involving these neighbours. My local newspaper ran an interview about my struggle for justice and the awful neighbours – who thankfully have since been evicted. There was silence from my psychiatrist. Of course, he didn't apologise. He is not a man of courage. He is happy with his nice little job looking after elderly people, and doesn't want any hassle from his patients. If I hadn't challenged him when I did, he would have simply increased my medication.

Fitness is an essential part of my mental and physical health, creating a secure foundation for alertness, energy and the strengthening of my will power. Before discovering exercise, the sky was darker, bolder with a hint of grey. The clouds zigzagged in motion. They appeared confused, as if not knowing which direction to turn. This resembled my mind, which was all over the place, longing for direction and a fulfilling purpose, but mostly just seeking peace. I believe exercise is particularly important for depression because inertia is at its very centre and makes people give up far too easily. Exercise makes me feel fitter, younger and healthier. Cycling is an excellent form of exercise for depression. I often cycle out into the countryside, which always has a good effect on my mood because it allows me to be present in the moment. I enjoy the beauty of the sun and the sky, while listening to birdsong and observing wild animals – which I find is a form of relaxation in itself. I've also discovered that indoor cardiovascular exercise on my rowing machine is important during wintertime, which is a particularly difficult time for depressives because of its bad weather and short, gloomy days. Last summer I returned to rowing after a break of fifty years and joined the local amateur rowing club which I now attend three times a week. It turned out to be one of the most demanding experiences of my life and also one of the most enjoyable. I go about my business of living with minor depressions all the time, but in addition to my exercise regime I am a member of a film club, as well as attending university society dinners. Parts of me are still at odds with myself, but I function. However, I find that actively pursuing a healthy lifestyle, working hard to stay fit and taking Lithium frees me from the extremes of bipolar.

Most people fail to recognise or understand the shame people with depression go through or how inadequate it makes them feel. The other taboo is sex. It is the first part of your being that disappears when you are depressed and then when manic it is the first arousal. I have always loved sex. Without wanting to sound like a born-again lothario, I have been married twice but society frowns on hearing that elderly people can enjoy satisfying sex lives into their seventies and beyond.

Is there a cure for bipolar? Well if there is, I haven't found it. The beginning of my troubles began when I was seven. The country was at war. My father was away working in a hospital. My mother struggled to cope with six children. And then the V1 bombs came down over Croydon, resulting in Winston Churchill's government coming up with an evacuation plan. It was made compulsory for every household in the country who had a spare room to take in war evacuees. I was split up from my mother and other siblings, leaving me and my sister, who was two years older, to be sent off to live with an elderly, childless couple in Somerset. They made it clear from the outset that we weren't wanted. Their house was cold. Their food was cold. A smile never dared to appear on their faces. Every breath of air had to be tinged with misery because otherwise their lungs would have rejected it. The old man continually stared at my sister, like he had never seen a young girl before, but he never looked at me. That was my first experience of loneliness and isolation. The feeling of abandonment has stayed with me all my life. When I look back I now realise that was indeed the first time I became depressed. I simply shut down. There are still times when I get flashbacks of back then. I can be in a room full of people when something occurs that sparks a memory of that time, leaving me frozen, unable to move. Experiences like this scar the consciousness and stay with you for your entire life.

For me, bipolar is something that I live with. I doubt there is a cure. You just have to develop a capacity to address it. It is a condition – a part of my life – but I have discovered ways to live with it through exercise, sex and intellectual pursuits. There are times that I am still mildly manic – but my wife is able to recognise any change in my usual personality and points it out to me that I am 'tripping'. I never get manic in an unpleasant way, but I become argumentative, like a dog with a bone. When this happens, my wife says to me, "For God's sake, just let it go."

Bipolar is like nature, which does not bloom all year round. Trees become alive with new growth in springtime, yet by autumn they are ready to shed their leaves once more. Summer is synonymous with warmth, beauty and fun, while winter illustrates our darker, colder and more foreboding character. You mustn't let bipolar run you, and neither should people shrug their shoulders and say, "I have no control over it." They, like me, like thousands of other ordinary people, need to learn ways to control it. It's not easy. If someone told me forty years ago how difficult it would be I wouldn't have believed them. But you have to get your life into perspective, you have to understand it, before you can accept and appreciate it for what it is. This is paramount if you are to get through the extremes of life, the ups and downs and run the gauntlet of emotions and experiences that come in between.

Summary of my life with bipolar:

1. I was diagnosed at eighteen but have often wondered if the diagnosis was accurate because I have rarely been really manic.

2. I am mostly prone to severe depressive episodes lasting weeks – then I become well again for several months. It is almost like I change with the seasons.

3. Both my parents and older sister are prone to depression, although none of them have official diagnoses and none of them ever seem to get as depressed as I do.

4. I am currently taking Valdoxan (Agomelatine) which is an antidepressant for severe depression – and Olanzapine (Zyprexa) which is an antipsychotic.

5. I'm unsure what caused being bipolar but I think an unstable family background when I was a child didn't help. Dad was in the army and we seemed to be forever moving home. Trouble with my sexuality contributed as my mother hated me for being gay.

6. I attempted suicide once in my late teens, because I too hated being gay – and sometimes still do.

7. I trust the medical profession fairly well and see my psychiatrist every three months.

8. I attended counselling on and off for six months. This helped me pull myself together and get a job. However, when I asked my psychiatrist if he could refer me for some more sessions he told me I couldn't have more than what I had already received. I think this was more the fault of the Irish health service than his.

9. I have managed to hold a job down for two years in a travel agency without too much difficulty.
10. I don't think my lifestyle is particularly healthy, as I smoke twenty cigarettes a day, but I also try to do thirty minutes of light exercise daily as well as walking to and from work.

Peter

Rita

*There is a lodger who comes and stays in my house –
sometimes for a couple of weeks and at other times for
several months. There is no set pattern of arrival – or
indeed season. Daffodils can be in full bloom or the
landscape can be covered with snow. Occasionally,
a year passes when without explanation she doesn't
visit. Often, people remark that she is like my shadow
because of her resemblance to me in appearance,
voice and how she reacts to situations. I dismiss
this comparison because I prefer to think of her as
a ghost – albeit a poor, fake, imitation ghost of me,
otherwise known as depression.*

*I often get asked what it feels like, being so depressed
that it makes me not want to leave my bedroom for
long periods. They don't know how easy it is to stay
in bed when you have lost all self-respect – when you
don't care about anything anymore – when you are
indifferent as to whether you live or die. It wouldn't
daunt me if the walls around me began to crack and
crumble. I would remain lying still – motionless but
without fear. Life can be painful and poignant, yet
I believe it to be precious and immeasurable. I keep
reminding myself that depression is only one part of
the larger story – and hope to see the day when this
ghost-like guest will leave and never return.*

My introduction to depression came early in life. Throughout my teenage years I was very unhappy, and during my early twenties I remember staying in bed for long periods. I found it difficult to be honest with myself, and to find the correct words to articulate the sensations of hopelessness, pain and suffering that were inside me. Searching for the correct word to convey the true nature of my feelings still seems to elude me, because a near enough description is not near enough at all. The feeling demands my efforts to find the right way to say what I need to say. This may sound like a non-starter, but if I cannot find the words to understand how desperate I feel, then how can I ever expect anyone else to understand what effect it is having on me? Although I didn't initially attribute this to depression, in hindsight I can see it bore the trademarks of my mother's illness. I'm convinced bipolar is genetic and that I stepped into my mother's shoes and became like her – depressed for several weeks at a time, intermingled with occasional elevated moods. Like her, I'm neither grandiose nor reckless when manic; rather I become obsessed with gardening and with cleaning the house, while surviving on little sleep.

Mental illness was a big stigma back when I was in my twenties. Although people speak more about it in the media these days, individual families still struggle with accepting it when it knocks on their own door. Even I was in denial for years, although I watched my mother go in and out of hospital numerous times during my youth. The fact is I was a parent long before I became a parent, having had to take on the role. My father died in a car crash when I was thirteen, and being an only child I had to assume responsibility of taking care of my mother when she became unwell. My aunt used to come and stay with me during those admissions, but I was the only one who went to visit her, which was always like the scene of a robbery with the sight of dejected faces on display in my mother's dormitory. It appeared as if their lust for life had been stolen. And then back at home, it was I who had to deal with the noisy neighbours, with one of them getting satisfaction every time she enquired, "Do you think she'll ever snap out of it?"

Indeed, my earliest memories of my mother are of her always being in bed. Just like me seeing my mother unwell, my son, too, will have seen similar scenes when he was young, when I stayed in bed for lengthy periods. I feel guilty about this but my mother didn't feel guilty because she was too wrapped up in her unhappiness to explain what was troubling her. I tried probing, but she found it difficult to relate to people. I'm the opposite; I love to talk about my feelings, but my husband isn't the easiest person to talk too. He's old stock – the type that can't show emotion or empathise with another person – or at least not in an open way. I've wanted him to understand me better but he always refuses to accompany me to medical appointments so that the doctor can explain. My son, too, also has this same reserved demeanour.

My latest serious bout of depression was after my niece died of cervical cancer. She was only thirty-four. It was an incredibly stressful time, watching her get weaker and weaker before she died, but also rewarding because I enjoyed helping to look after her, as it gave me a purpose. But I know that, subconsciously, I must have become too absorbed in her suffering by the depth of my loneliness and heartache afterwards. I'm good at looking after sick people. As well as having taken care of my mother, I worked in a care home for elderly nuns, which was a bit of an eye-opener. The nuns were unkind to each other despite many of them being frail. There was a hierarchical rule amongst them which meant that those who had been teachers wouldn't speak to those who had worked in the kitchen or laundry. I had lost my faith years earlier, not because of this experience but owing to the clerical abuse scandals that have eaten away at the Catholic Church in the last twenty years like a moth that eats a piece of cloth bit by bit until a hole appears in its fabric. Being unable to share my feelings with my husband or son left me in a black hole – complete with a spiritual emptiness. But just before my niece died, a young American priest came into the hospice and gave her the last rights. He then laid his hands on my head and gave me a blessing. It was like I was pining for him to come along and then one day he arrived by chance. There was something in the tone of his voice, in the warmth of the gentle words he expressed, which helped to re-ignite my faith. I'm convinced this made the sadness easier to endure in the darker moments after her death – and although I didn't start going to Mass again, I believe it prevented me from slipping too deeply into the depressive episode that followed.

I keep fighting and pushing myself to get better. I have come to terms with having bipolar as best I can. It's a question of making sure I get up every day and do things. I have osteoporosis and need to be careful not to fall or break any bones. I've started going to exercise classes and am considering taking up Tai Chi, which I'm told is a great way of keeping the body lucid. I take a mild sleeping tablet to stop me lying awake because the silence in the middle of the night is a lonely one. Then there is my main medication – 400mg of Lithium nightly. I'm also prescribed antidepressants but I no longer take them because they weren't working. My bedside table is littered with medication bottles, which I keep for reassurance should I become unwell again. There is no shortage of medication locally because we have our fair share of pharmaceutical companies – and factories too – where tablets are manufactured at low cost. Psychiatrists and chemists profit out of this arrangement. I've read in newspapers how they get free holidays to promote the products!

I am open to new ideas and have just heard about a support group in a neighbouring town for people with depression and other emotional issues, including bipolar. At the moment, I don't know anyone else with bipolar so it would be nice to hear how it affects others. I'm sure there will be people there who, like me, have nobody to confide in, so it will be good to give and receive support. I recently heard a man on my local radio station talking about mental health and depression. He recommended taking up Transcendental Meditation. The technique is based on Hindu Traditions for relaxing and refreshing the mind and body through the silent repetition of a special formula of words. I think it takes about six months to learn. I am open to new ideas and have become a great believer in alternative medicine. I am very optimistic about being cured. Having a future without Lithium takes priority in my life. I am sure there is an answer beyond psychiatric medication but I know a person needs strong willpower to find it. Patrick Holford engrossed me from the moment I first saw him on the Late Late Show. His book, The Feel Good Factor, made me think differently about my health and what I could do to improve my situation. I looked at his website and found it so interesting. There is a section devoted to bipolar which looks at nutritional imbalances and outlines an action plan that entails adding Omega 3 fats to your diet as well as reducing caffeine, sugar and alcohol.

I plan to go to Holford's next seminar in Cork and am slowly changing my diet after becoming more conscious about food supplements. I have been using a lot of mixtures of nuts, seeds and Omega 3 and 6 sprinkled on my breakfast cereal. I am also taking daily starflower and fish oil capsules. Holford also recommends 5HTP to relax and to get to sleep – and marine oil, which is good for producing serotonin. Sunshine is not very plentiful where I live, and he also suggests exercise with plenty of fresh air, which is hard to achieve when depression sets in, so I always make sure I walk a mile every day. Right now I am in a good place. I am calm and feeling happier about my life. An aura of contentment and hope has taken a gentle hold, making me look towards the future more than at any other point in my life.

Daniel

When I'm depressed, my entire attention is focused on this state every waking moment of the day. I suffer from insomnia, so my days are long and it further compounds my struggle with depression when I haven't slept. I have no energy and am constantly tired but this doesn't stop my mind berating me and telling me that I'm not good enough, not fast enough. I fear unfamiliarity and hate being around strangers or being placed in situations in which I have to express myself. It is a little like having a broken leg in the sense that you can stand up but you fear walking. But I push myself to function at a level where I can live my life doing the things I love – writing, filmmaking and graphic art.

> *I Tai Chi my way through the day*
> *Taekwondo through the afternoon*
> *Shadow box through the evening*
> *And Karate through the night*
> *But my muscles aren't enough*
> *While I yoga the sun set in my mind*
> *I'm a tree, I'm a crane, I'm cloud*
> *But it's not enough in depression's shroud.*

I was twenty-eight when my brother killed himself. I am still haunted by the image of him hanging there, his body limp and listless, broken by a ruthless dumb rope that was incapable of leniency. I'm now on my twelfth different antidepressant in the nine years since he died. I feel better some days than others, unhappy but not melancholic. I maintain a measure of calm and can feign contentment in order to please others and be accepted by them. Maybe that's one of the reasons I'm easily placated by my doctor. We exchange a few superficial words about the medication not working. "Trial by error," he says, before changing my prescription again. I once tried counselling with a psychoanalyst. She told me I had her total trust, resulting in me confiding in her fully. But then she suddenly cancelled our next appointment and a short time later, I received a letter saying she had left the practice. I felt I had wasted my time and effort and couldn't bring myself to seek out a new therapist because I didn't want to start at the beginning again and have to explain my life story to someone new.

At first they listened with mind control
Prescribed a diet of medicine in kind
chemicals etch lines on glass of the soul
Acting as a pillow choking the mind
Like bad grammar drugs talking with my voice
Brain pesticides as razors whisper gently
to the veins, can't feel, can't hurt, what choice
this migraine of hurt smiles indifferently
Silenced by candied saints such works of art
thoughts drain away in shadows of deep red
the floor drinks the ink from the heart
Asked for help instead drugs we were fed.
Think you're clever now just as dead as ever

I can still see their faces and smell their perfume. Their crying grew louder and louder as I entered the room. It felt like I was intruding upon their grief, tiptoeing around them, yet at the same time unable to understand why I wasn't able to cry whilst their tears flowed freely. I was twelve when my father died suddenly from a heart attack. There are moments even now when I grasp for breath when I recall leaning into the coffin to kiss him goodbye and feeling his cold skin against my lips. For a long time afterwards I couldn't bear to be around too many people. I'm quite neurotic, really. The sound of a radio in the background, a television being too loud or a dog barking irritates me, and often I respond in cantankerous tones. I still find it difficult to react to stressful situations, hence my acute depressive episodes and 'burn outs'.

> *Bowing down crazy tenebrous beauty*
> *beating lullabies in my chest*
> *dizzying parliaments of thought*
> *crucified against a wall of wordings*
> *divided sentiments in protraction*
> *marble mantels where calla lilies sleep*
> *battle sovereign tearless sadness*
> *suffering stylish grace of darling sorrow*
> *hammering inside ever faster*
> *died on my feet, dying while walking*
> *cried can't run, can't run away,*
> *demon's hoof crushes my throat*
> *havens in silly paper bag aren't enough*

It's like a root that grows within me and is determined by the seasons. I can remain depressed for periods lasting as long as four months. During these times I am extremely tired and when placed in hyper-stressful situations I am unable to make simple decisions, resulting in me having to struggle desperately for an answer each time. My family understand what I going through when this happens and have preserved my sanity during these episodes by listening, making me know how much they care. I find depression has its good points though. Unlike mania, it has become a silent friend that slows me down and provides powerful introspective moments where I can plot great story lines such as delving into the horrors of famines and wars, as well as searching life for moments of great beauty and grace, whilst exploring the mysteries of God and the universe.

You're nailed in my heart
Haunting my thoughts
flames ignited in my eyes
I hate you but I love you
No rain upon my soul
Burning in the night
A beast clawing in my veins
I hate you but I love
Like an angel on fire
I've drunk your anger
In the ruins of Eden
I hate you but I love
So diving into the dark
I can't love you but I do
It was me you marked
Next door in my mind
Tedious moments within
Such chemical boredom
I hate you but I love you

Sometimes a mist comes over me and I wonder what it would feel like to die. I close my eyes and in a trance-like state imagine my spirit floating away from my body. It's not that I want to die or ever have any intention of killing myself. It's the opposite really, because I have discovered no matter how depressed I am it won't last. Likewise, no matter how high my moods reach, they too will evolve into another state. My support mechanisms are good. My valued friends kindly ask me how I'm feeling but I dare not bore them too much with my woes. But I occasionally make a mistake and know I have done so when one of them says, "You've talked about this before." I used to have the habit of laboriously going over the same problem, time after time, but I've stopped doing that. Thankfully no one abandoned me on this account, but I have learned to be careful of the possibility.

Shadows swell in the dark
The sword is blade heavy
And the shield is broken
Lonely behind armour
Dwelling on but one knee
Black in a starless sky
Rebellion in the mists
The soul gently falls down
Cimmerian sadness
Where pale eyed wolves whisper
A Knight with no castle
lonely beyond belief

My problem is I think too hard. In my least creative moments I get ocular migraines because of pressure on my optic nerve.

Boredom challenges my sanity and comes after there's been a lull in my life, usually caused by a change of pace after I've finished a project. Other times I wish I could take my brain out of my head and clean it like a plate gets cleaned in a dishwasher. But on whole I am happy with all the variety my life offers and more importantly I appreciate that I alone am in charge of my destiny. My decisions are entirely mine and equally my mistakes belong to me too. This philosophy works for me but even if it didn't, I believe life has a way of pushing you along regardless. Nothing stays the same forever. I wish suicidal people could realise this. Anyone can die if they want to. Suicide is hardly an achievement. No, the real achievement is to stay put and push through the hurdles to a point where you end up appreciating your life for what it is.

> *Portions of death I eat each day.*
> *Yet only a cup full of fear I drink.*
> *Little men with hammers strike my mind,*
> *they all have names; Boredom and Sanity*
> *And their cousin Mania drills in my head.*
> *The debris of their work weighs me down,*
> *what I would give for a spring-clean!*
> *Lancing the dragon of pain*
> *welcoming the morning star.*
> *Is this the birth of another terrible day?*
> *Or for once will my burden fall away?*

Darkness and light exist along with each other quite amicably. Memories never go away but it is up to everyone to analyse their thoughts and to accept what has happened in their past. I had a girlfriend once and I listened to her problems, gave advice and at one point wanted to protect her from all her suffering. But during the process I soaked up the sadness of her pain. I realised we were not good for each other and took a step back. I equated myself to someone who had just stopped smoking and had started a relationship with someone who was a heavy smoker. The temptation to smoke was intense. In our case, we provided ammunition to each other to dwell constantly on our problems – and that was something I knew wasn't healthy to do.

There is sadness still within my eyes
I've needed something to hold onto
Just a moment's pause before it dies
This grey and blackness obscures your view
Fewer blooms upon the phoenix tree
No tears just a silence as it waits
It's fine, release your ache upon my chest
Sorrow twists, biting barbs, as it grates
Within my arms you were once at rest
Death doesn't require camaraderie
soaked up all your pain with my heart
Much is unimportant, yes it's true
You know my soul like a faded chart
Just a dim shadow now without you
It calls me, the voice of the banshee
Eternity was never meant to be
Just pop another pill, it's ok I'm always with you

I recognised it every time I looked at my mother's face and could feel her hurt and read the pain in her eyes, knowing her soul grieved for my father and brother. The joy of life has diminished from her. I felt impossibly useless by not being able to comfort her but at the same time excused myself from any duty. I now realise the same is happening to me and there is nothing I want to do about it. Depression and mania are what makes me. I'd feel lost without them, like bereavement − so to make sure I never lose them, I have instead normalised them into my existence. It is *I* who has created this life − and *I* who must be content with my creation by lying on the bed I have made.

This unreachable hurt
holding my breath
waiting, counting, hoping
this little death

Silences are painful
barbed wire around my mind
waiting, trying, still hoping
alone with shadows in kind

Hammers on an anvil of angels
crippled by a creeping dread
not waiting no longer hoping
Standing up lonely and dead
My soul hurts in longing
memories ache my conscience
Just tired of wishing
This painful melody in silence
Tick tock, unbreathing

tock tick, still dying
The clock mocks, the clock ticks
Warning, choking, sobbing

I can't stop hurting.

I sometimes gaze at my hands and fingers, mesmerised by how strange I think they look. Simple objects can seem extraordinary. I once stared at my bedroom door for hours, baffled at its existence. I wondered how old the timber was, dissecting every notch and examining in minute detail its creation and relevance – while also being transfixed by its metal hinges, screws and handle. I imagined the door had intestines and wanted to imagine what they looked like. I closed my eyes to do this, but thankfully fell asleep instead, exhausted after days without sleep.

Distant echoing of a heart in yesterday's sun
The light must again shine through the rain
Somewhere is a place for us where we can run
Perfumed rage pulses in delicate veins

Lost in glass affection shimmer and fall
tomorrow's anger is just another day
More difficult to say nothing at all
farewell's embrace is yet another way

still hearing their whispering voices
rescue what may from that bitter moon
The last chance we have as is our choice
listening over and over to the same old tune.

In perfect loneliness I dwelt in the aftermath
Plaster-of-Paris encases my heart with pills
I dwell now in the beauty of another path
light reflects peaceful tears of yet more ills.
The mist pillows my soul like a place I knew
Drifting towards rainbows over distant waterfalls
home near the mountains where warmer winds blew
Even medicine has its most beautiful flaws.

After the rain has stopped, the sun comes out, but depression becomes mundane. It is like an old, familiar visitor who bores you and yet needs rejuvenation, something I needed when another relationship failed. Over the years my doctor insisted on increasing my antidepressants, which in hindsight was a disastrous plan. The extra medication robbed me of the ability to feel emotion; numbing my thoughts and making me feel dead inside, an empty heart that became more frozen after each dosage. I sometimes wonder why psychiatrists don't account for the inability of medication to help people reflect on their mistakes or to resolve difficulties. If I am in a relationship in the future that breaks down, I will try hard not to take extra medication to quash whatever turmoil I'm experiencing and will let my heart heal at its own pace.

There is dirt in my blood
The weirdness of mundanity
And tired prosaic little things
Haunted by thoughts
And harassed by insomnia
Running out of strength to fight you
I keep the vigil on the battlements

Watching for the weaknesses
I can't hold here by myself
But I'm all that's left of me
Leather wings and demonic things
An atomic bomb of fright springs
Hold my breath, count and count
Picked up my lance the dragon's eye
Breathe out, here it comes
I can't retreat any further
Time to live or time to die
None see the battle waged
While I take the elevator to hell.

Sometimes, nature is neither attractive nor calm. Like a summer thunderstorm, you can smell the distinctive scent of rain after it has stopped. Later, when the scent diminishes, you know it will return but not until similar levels of heat have occurred again – and there is nothing you can do but wait and be prepared. At least I have the assurance I survived the storm before and that I will survive it again. So that's my life, whether you consider it sad, interesting, boring or dreary. I've learned I am the author of my script and that I need to be the hero of my story. I haven't given up hope that one day my personal storm will clear and I'll be able to see far over a clear horizon. When this happens, I'll write another script and give it a happier ending.

Part 3

Being Fully Informed

Introduction

We live in an age when it has never been easier to find information. In a shrinking world, anyone with a computer and an internet connection can find information on anything, from the sex life of dung beetles to the formation of stars.

But information in itself is not power. *Knowledge* is power – the ability to sift through the waves and waves of data and understand what is relevant and useful, and what is merely factual detritus or misinformation.

In this information age, then, it has also never been more important to control the story. To guide the perceptions of those seeking information the way you want them to go. In the age of advertising, controlling buzz-words and phrases is the key to what your audience understands. 'Chemical imbalance' is a case in point. Pharmaceutical companies and Big Psychiatry sell psychotropic drugs and cures the way other industries sell washing powder. "Holistic, non-drug therapies may leave your psyche looking grubby and unhealthy. Opt for new UberLithium, and get your mental processes really clean..."

The example may seem flippant, but the point is valid: alternative therapies which don't put money in the pockets of Big Pharma and Big Psychiatry are belittled, ridiculed and have no access to the kind of funding or marketing that the drug options do. Doctors routinely prescribe drug treatments as a first response, and certainly within an overstretched NHS, complex conditions like bipolar are reduced to a symptom-list and auto-treated with drugs. And the principles of patient care have been co-opted by the twin pillars of Big Psychiatry and Big Pharma.

It is not the purpose of this book to actively recommend alternative treatments. I am not a doctor, and nor do I claim any medical knowledge. But opening the minds of readers to non-drug treatments as possible aids to their healing and management seems entirely valid here. This is offered in the interests of redressing the knowledge-balance of patients who may not even be aware that such non-drug therapies exist, let alone what kind of successes they have been shown to have.

I have contacted many people working in alternative areas for workable solutions, and while I have taken much time to research for factual evidence, I am not responsible for the comments, ideas or beliefs of the writers and health professionals quoted in this book.

What follows in this chapter is a sample (not by any means a definitive list) of alternative, drug-free treatments and therapies, covering the main areas that lead to optimum good health and recovery from bipolar.

One thing though is clear: change is never delivered from above – it must be made at grass roots level. From the moment you receive a diagnosis of bipolar, you will be on the conveyor belt of drug and in some cases electro treatments. If you want to get off the conveyor belt, you cannot wait for the medical or psychiatric professions to suggest alternatives – it's not in their interests. You have to be pro-active in seeking the alternatives that work for you: after all, it's your life.

Self-Management

Remember, bipolar disorder is a condition of two extremes. Although timescales vary between individuals, there will be periods of mania that last one to four weeks when the person's moods become elevated and they experience high energy levels with little need for sleep. They will become uninhibited and be prone to risk-taking, which can be coupled with bouts of anxiety and paranoia. Manic episodes will be followed by periods of depression lasting six months or shorter, in which the person spends most of the day in bed, coupled with little motivation or interest to do anything in life, including a lack of desire to even eat. There will be long periods of remission in between manic and depressive episodes. And then there will be times during this period when the person is slightly elevated but not manic – and likewise with the depression, when the person is slightly low but can cope with daily life.

It is paramount that the cause of the highs and lows is identified. It is no good considering the symptoms to be the main problem because in reality they are just masking the cause – and although the exact cause of bipolar remains unknown, the answer just might likely lie in one of the following:

- A traumatic event in your life and how it affected your emotions.
- Are you affected by poor nutrition?

- Misuse of drugs or alcohol – or both.
- Undiagnosed medical conditions.
- Are there deficiencies in minerals and vitamins?
- Are there unnecessary and dangerous toxins in your system?
- Perhaps organic causes need to be explored?
- What about lead poisoning or other heavy metals?
- Are there problems in the central nervous system?
- What about abnormalities in the DNA structure?
- Have you had vaccinations recently?
- Have you come into contact with pesticides or chemical sprays?

We need to look at safe, natural solutions instead of resorting first and foremost to psychiatric medication. There are no magic solutions, rather only ones that require time, willpower and commitment to achieve. Recovery is primarily based on a good healthy lifestyle consisting of a sensible diet, exercise, sleep and the absence of drug and alcohol misuse. Effective coping skills can be developed through insight into the condition; a support network of friends is helpful, perhaps also talking therapies – and for some, religious and spiritual practice.

This chapter looks at a few of the many other workable solutions, some of which are outside of medical psychiatric practices. These are not designed to be definitive answers, but I believe from the professionals I have consulted with that they are a sound basis from which to start the healing journey, particularly if you are looking for solutions without the need for psychiatric drugs – or at the very least lessening your need for such drugs. I believe that the more information and answers you gather, the more likely you are to making an informed choice about your health and treatment.

Bipolar is not unlike a physical condition, in that you can help by managing unnecessary stimulation of the problem. Nobody knows a person better than the person themself. Therefore, someone with bipolar will need to equip themself with new strategies to monitor moods. For some, this will entail moving away from a life of dependency and moving towards taking charge of their own destiny. In order for change to occur they will need to develop awareness that certain factors increase anxiety, hyperactivity, stress and depression. Some of these pitfalls include:

- stressful situations in work and relationships that cause emotional strain and anxiety
- working exceptionally long hours
- insufficient sleep
- having a bad diet
- a lifestyle with no exercise
- misusing alcohol and recreational drugs (either cannabis or other illicit substances).

I recommend people keep a daily journal and write down thoughts, feelings and behaviours as this will help develop awareness to variations in mood patterns. Managing anxiety means a regular sleep pattern and lifestyle changes to help combat anxiety and depression as listed above. In addition I would also recommend the following:

- Go for a walk and see how a stroll for half an hour in your local neighbourhood or nearby park can be therapeutic.
- Clean up your environment – a spring clean of your home and a sort out of correspondence, bills and official documentation may help.
- Maintain a social network by staying in touch with friends – by telephone, text or email and arrange to meet up. Other ways of improving communication is to use social network sites like Facebook or join a social group or night class that will help develop new friendships.
- Try some new relaxation technique – for example yoga, which is designed to help reduce anxiety and promote harmony of mind and body. It is a great way to be gentle with yourself.
- Think about the future. Get three sheets of paper and mark them past, present and future. On the first sheet of paper, write down the key events of your past. On the second sheet, list events going on in your life at present. The future can sometimes feel like a blank sheet of paper. We can learn from the past as it provides us with wisdom but it doesn't have to determine our future – unless we allow it to. Therefore, on the third sheet of paper list your plans, hopes and goals for the future, no matter how small because these will grow and develop with perseverance.
- I would recommend a book called *Alternatives Beyond Psychiatry*, co-edited by Peter Lehmann and

Peter Stastny, which is written by authors, ex-users and survivors of psychiatry, therapists, psychiatrists, social scientists, lawyers and relatives – who are all in agreement that society needs to go beyond psychiatry and the current concept of 'mental illness', which is a stumbling block towards looking at other viable, working alternatives.

Ultimately, a good understanding of how to manage the symptoms before they escalate is essential in managing this condition. So be adventurous and don't be unwilling to try out new things or shift patterns in your way of thinking about your life and how you live it.

Mood Stabilising Medications

Throughout this chapter, readers are encouraged to take a different look at their lives and how they treat their bodies. Instead of reaching out first and foremost for medication to alleviate their distress, which in turn leads to long-term health problems and addiction, I want people to be fully informed, because I believe people can be cured. I believe people should be fully informed about treatments and should be made aware of all treatment options. The following pages are some of the many alternatives offered to me through my research and provide a comprehensive list of ideas, showing alternative methods available which address the causes rather than just treating the symptoms.

In several cases certain medications have a place in the foundation of treatment for bipolar, for example, when someone is in the initial throes of mania, a tranquillising drug may be the only option to use at that time, but only for a short period of time (less than a week) to avoid trauma and stress to the patient because long-term use can attack the central nervous system and become addictive.

My research has led me to believe that the following may be beneficial in such instances:

- Low dosage of antipsychotics when the person is experiencing a severe manic episode (older types seems to be the safest and best – fewer side-effects and less addictive) or a low dosage of immunosystem drugs/autonomic drugs.

- EPA or Eicosapentaenoic acid is an essential Omega 3 fatty acid. It is essential to take because the body cannot synthesise this by itself, and therefore needs to obtain it from dietary sources. EPA fish oil has been shown to markedly improve mood disorders helping people feel less depressed, balanced and stable.

Once the person has gained some control over their manic episode they can begin the process of identifying the underlying cause. If it is trauma caused by a life event, consideration should be given to perhaps counselling, homeopathy, diet and exercise. If there is a physical cause, this should be tended to like any other illness would be treated with conventional medicine.

Unlike mania, where short-term medication can be used, the use of antidepressants in the first instances of periods of depression is not advised. Antidepressants can sometimes increase the risk of developing suicidal thoughts (and even committing suicide) so the need to look at safer, more effective options is paramount and I believe the key to this is homeopathy (which is featured in this chapter). I fully acknowledge that depression is hard to 'snap' out of, but instead of going to your GP or psychiatrist, I believe people should be encouraged to be open to other options – to prevent becoming addicted to tablets that can in some cases ruin their health and will not cure their depression, but often make it worse and could make them suicidal. It is essential that the underlying cause of disturbed sleep, loss of energy and physical aches and pains is established.

Depression comes on gradually, with the sufferer not always aware of what is happening. Family and friends are usually the first to notice that there's a problem. Here, people need to become better educated to encourage sufferers of depression to seek out what is really causing the depression rather than depending on their GP or psychiatrist and accept the sometimes-easiest option of being prescribed antidepressants. Serotonin is primarily found in the gastrointestinal tract, platelets, and in the central nervous system, and is a contributor to feelings of well-being and happiness. Ask your doctor for a serotonin blood test to measure the amount of serotonin in your body.

Explore other natural solutions because there are many available, for example:

- Have you considered counselling to get to the root of the problem?
- Be willing to explore homeopathy, aromatherapy or reflexology. The latter can particularly help with sleep problems as the practitioner works on the pituitary gland, which controls sleep patterns in the brain.
- Outdoor exercise in daylight will help enormously to break people of the cycle of poor motivation and inertia.
- Pay a visit to your local health store and get 5-HTP natural amino acid capsules – which support a normal mood, healthy nervous system and serotonin production.
- Acupuncture is also known to release serotonin.

- Examine your diet – fruits with a good ratio of serotonin include dates, papayas and bananas – also eating a diet low in carbohydrates and high in protein will increase serotonin by secreting insulin, which helps in amino acid balance.

Withdrawing from medication

People with mental health problems are treated as a minority group and thus often live in a human rights ghetto. People need to start realising that they have a right to have a say about what drugs go into their body, so never hesitate to ask for your medication to be reviewed with the proviso that it gets reduced over a supervised period of time. This will open up the opportunity to introduce other treatments (which I shall discuss later in this chapter).

I cannot emphasise enough how highly addictive antipsychotic, antidepressants and mood stabilising medications can be – and how difficult it is to be weaned off them because of the severe withdrawal symptoms. It is not unlike withdrawing from illicit street drugs owing to the reaction within the central nervous system when the drugs leave the bloodstream. Coming off psychotropic drugs may produce the following withdrawal symptoms:

- aggression
- dizziness
- vomiting
- headaches
- depression
- suicidal tendencies.

Sudden withdrawal can make some people suddenly become acutely unwell because of falling levels of the drugs in the bloodstream. Several texts warn of this danger: Moore (1998), Tubridy and Corry (2001) and Glenmullen (2006) all outline how it is essential that withdrawal is done under strict medical supervision. This may appear easier said than done because many psychiatrists will be reluctant or even refuse to help their patients achieve this goal. But any person who really wants to withdraw should not be deterred by this. They can seek a private psychiatrist who may assist or alternatively, if this is not possible, they should consider contacting a mental health users group for advocacy or seek legal advice or contact a human rights organisation. Frankly, nothing is impossible because where there is a will there will always be a way.

Drugs must be slowly reduced in order for the body to replenish its own levels of natural resources, because otherwise cells within the central nervous system will react to the sudden withdrawal of the drugs. This entails a reverse reaction to when the person first started taking the drugs in the first place. Initially, the cells go into shock when foreign receptors invade them, and although the body eventually adjusts to the psychotropic drugs, the drugs nevertheless silently continue to damage cells and in turn the person's immune system. However, sudden withdrawal confuses the cells, causing the body to react in a defiant manner against itself because the central nervous system mistakes the body's own natural resources as further foreign receptors.

When withdrawing from psychotropic drugs it is not uncommon for the person to become acutely unwell and to mirror symptoms of bipolar by having a manic episode with psychotic features followed by deep depression. While withdrawing from the drugs must be done under medical supervision, I am under no illusion of how difficult this might be for some patients who are both addicted to them and fear becoming unwell if they cease medication. There will also be the fear of approaching your psychiatrist with the view of reduction leading to total cessation, because as you will have seen in the *Life Stories*, arguing with a psychiatrist is a daunting prospect. Challenging them is fearful because you know the power they have and perhaps have experienced the full wrath of this if ever you have been sectioned under the Mental Health Act. Can anything be more terrifying than having your civil liberty taken away, being fed drugs against your will, being told lies and myths about your 'illness', none more so than that you will have to take medication for the rest of your life in order to combat your mental problem?

Some guidance points to coming off medication must include the following:

1. Ask yourself whether you are ready to come off the medication. Do you feel confident enough for the challenges ahead? Have you read up on the facts, so that you are making an informed choice? Have you discussed it with your family and doctor?

2. The initial dosage reduction must be small, no more that 25%, to avoid becoming acutely unwell.

3. You must work alongside your doctor who will monitor withdrawal symptoms and advise accordingly – or find a competent practitioner who can assist you.

4.   You must wait for additional reductions until your doctor recommends them, which will be based on your withdrawal symptoms and the time required for these to alleviate.

5.   A final medical examination should be done after you have completely stopped taking all drugs – with lifestyle changes made that embrace alternative methods to maintain good health, both physically and mentally.

Finally, there is a book that I would like to recommend entitled *Psychiatric Drug Withdrawal: A Guide for Prescribers, Therapists, Patients and families* by Dr Peter Breggin (2012). This fully describes what steps to take to get off psychotropic drugs. It also calls for psychiatric nurses, psychologists and social workers to become better educated on these harmful drugs and to stop pushing their clients to take them – and not to dictate to clients how long they must stay on them. There is also a good website worth looking at **www.alternativetomeds.com** Although, this is an American site, it will illustrate how there are ways of achieving a drug free life. This website may give you some ideas, thereby planting seeds that will enable you to seek an alternative treatment to psychiatric drugs.

Medical Examinations

Some people have a family GP who knows their entire medical history – but this won't be the case for others who move to a new area or those living in large towns and cities and who experience frequent changes. And yet, as previously mentioned, the GP surgery is so often the place where peoples' psychiatric journeys begin – where antidepressants are readily prescribed after a minimal few minutes of discussion without any extensive medical examinations or tests being carried out. It is essential to start at the beginning and ask the question, 'Why?' because pain and suffering can manifest themselves in many different ways, for example, an overactive thyroid gland has been seen to mimic the symptoms of bipolar. Brain injuries can occur in people through falls, sporting injuries, fights and road accidents, particularly in young people and this often results in erratic behaviour and depression. Therefore, it is advised that any physical underlying condition is located and identified, which otherwise could manifest itself as a so-called mental illness. The only way to achieve this is through a full and searching medical examination.

We are complex individuals. There isn't one simple solution to explain the underlying cause of emotional distress, but firstly you have got to eliminate what it's 'not'. Do not accept the lie that you have a chemical imbalance of the brain or that you have a genetic illness over which you have no control, unless you wish to be destined for a lifetime of medication.

You must also be aware that your doctor may not be well trained in nutrition and its effects on the body – after all she/he is a doctor of 'medicine' and not a doctor of nutrition. So any information you can provide from doing your own research into your symptons on the internet may be of great importance in getting his cooperation in doing the necessary tests. Alternatively, you may want to seek out doctors who are trained in nutritional and allergy testing. You have the right to insist that your doctor helps you to find that underlying cause. In any event, a doctor must be prepared to take into account the welfare of the person in front of them by means of a battery of tests including examinations for:

- allergies
- toxins
- exposure to chemicals.

Further tests may include:

- blood
- urine
- hair/nail
- tests for vitamin or mineral deficiencies.

It may also be necessary to have either an MRI scan or X-ray.

- MRI Scan – Magnetic Resonance Imaging is a medical test that helps doctors diagnose medical conditions, as well as it being the most sensitive image test carried out on the head and brain. An MRI scan helps produce detailed pictures of organs, soft tissues, bone and nearly all other internal body structures. It is able to detect brain tumours, infections, developmental anomalies, haemorrhage in trauma patients, chronic conditions such as multiple sclerosis, as well as disorders of the pituitary gland.

- X-ray – this is used to eliminate fractures or other physical damage to the brain or skeleton.

The body functions like a machine. A life span is 0–85 years on average with oxygen, vitamins, minerals, carbon dioxide, and proteins fuelling the body. If there are insufficient quantities of these, the body registers a deficiency and automatically reverts to being an engine that isn't functioning properly.

It is unfortunate that some GPs are poorly trained in mental health matters and will often go for the easiest option of prescribing antidepressants rather than looking for causes.

GPs operate under *NICE* guidelines, meaning they are trained to treat the presenting problems – in other words treat the symptoms that the patient is experiencing. But this is not good enough. It's your health we are talking about here. You want to find out what is causing your emotional distress. Tell them that you want to get to the real cause of what is wrong with you. Alert them to the fact that you are aware that you require a thorough examination to eliminate various potential physical causes.

Don't underestimate your own sense of awareness of what may or may not be right with you. Often you inherently know what is wrong and you should insist that the doctor gives you tests that you need.

If the main presenting problem is depression you must ask about access to counselling services, instead of the GP automatically reaching for the prescription pad.

More time and more effort are required. What's wrong with expecting that and not the customary 10 minutes currently available to each patient per visit? However, if your GP is unable or unwilling to carry out some tests or refer you for counselling, then please seek a practitioner who is willing to do what is being asked.

There are many centres, both in the UK and Ireland, that can assist you in seeking the appropriate tests and/or treatment and support and all of these and many others can be looked up on the internet:

- Breakspear Hospital in Hertfordshire
  www.breakspearmedical.com
- The Brain Bio Centre in London
  www.foodforthebrain.org
- Gut and Psychology practitioners – in both the UK and Ireland **www.gaps.me**
- Royal London Hospital of Homeopathy Medicine
  www.rlhh.eu
- The College of Naturopathic Medicine
  www.naturopathy-uk.com
- Critical Voices Network in Dublin
  www.criticalvoicesnetwork.com
- The Wellbeing Foundation in County Wicklow
  www.wellbeingfoundation.com
- MindFreedom Ireland
  www.mindfreedomireland.com
- MindFreedom UK **www.mindfreedom.org**

We are all responsible for ensuring we take good care of ourselves and that extends to the care and treatment of our bodies when we get sick. We should be very alert to a doctor who reaches too quickly for a prescription pad without doing the necessary medical or physical tests to determine his diagnosis. You should never be afraid to question a diagnosis or to seek a second opinion or look for alternative solutions. Remember, the doctor doesn't always know best!

Some thoughts on Suicide

There are no accurate statistics that collect information pertaining to suicide and those who kill themselves while on medication, but one questions how many people who kill themselves were taking antidepressants or antipsychotics at the time of their death? For many people with bipolar, these mind-altering tablets are the first in-road that leads to their depression – exacerbating rather than abating – and to more entrenched despair than would otherwise been experienced. People look for a way to end their lives because suicide is not a side-effect of antidepressants, it can be the *effect*. Suddenly a person is faced with the biggest crisis in his or her life. It becomes bigger than any period of desperation they have ever experienced before. It is also more profound than any problem they have previously sought an answer to, which turns into despair on such a scale that death is the only answer. But is there anything that can be done to reasonably prevent someone from killing themselves in an age in which antidepressants are freely prescribed and when access to harmful suicide-related websites is so easy?

Some key points to consider:

- The simple act of communication can never be underestimated and this is the key when dealing with people who are suicidal. Psychiatric evaluations are notorious for being opinionated rather than scientific. Patients will be told they have a chemical imbalance of the brain. Ask the person what they were told and then enquire what tests were done to verify an imbalance? There aren't any, so discrediting the falsehoods can have an immense impact on the person's mental outlook.

- Even if they had not been to see a psychiatrist or a doctor, I would ask them to tell me what was troubling them in the same vein that a friend would listen to a troubled associate. Ask them what has been/is going on in his/her life that is troubling them. Unlike a psychiatrist or a psychologist, I would not pass comment on what they told me, I would simply listen. Getting a person to talk is extremely therapeutic. You can also direct them to a reputable organisation like the Samaritans for support.

- Ask the person what mental illness or disorder they were diagnosed with and then direct them to data published by a reputable source that details the unscientific nature of psychiatric diagnoses. Recognising the fraudulent nature of psychiatric labels can assist a person, as it dispels what was otherwise accepted as truth. I have found a very extensive website that addresses the side-effects of psychiatric drugs and those commonly prescribed for bipolar compiled by the Citizens Commission on Human Rights: **www.cchrint.org**

- The next step is to recommend advice from a non-psychiatric medical practitioner and to undergo a battery of medical tests (not psychological assessments or evaluations) to find any undiagnosed physical conditions that could be manifesting as a so-called mental illness. It is a matter of sound medical fact that undiagnosed physical illness or injury can trigger emotional difficulties. Several studies over several decades – Fras et al. (1967), Hall et al. (1978) and Sternberg (1986) – have all shown that those diagnosed with mental illnesses were actually suffering from a physical condition. Suggesting this route of course depends on the emotional stability of the person. If they are in a position to assimilate information, direct them to a couple of websites that might be of assistance, such as the *Brain Bio Centre* in London **www.foodforthebrain.org** which was mentioned earlier in Medical Examinations and *The Road Back Programme* which gives practical advice on how to come off psychoactive drugs safely. **www.theroadback.org**

• If the person is taking a cocktail of psychiatric drugs, ask them what has been prescribed. Based on their reply, I would look up the details of the drugs on the British National Formulary (BNF) website **www.bnf.org** to see what effects were listed. Equally, I would ask the person to check the Patient Information Leaflet (PIL) to see what effects are also mentioned. A lot of psychiatric drugs have paradoxical effects*, such as suicidal ideation. Does the person know this? Were they informed at the point of the consultation? What did the prescriber tell them? I would explore this to find out what was said, and to find out exactly what information and understanding the person has. This is part of directing them along avenues where you are assisting them in finding the answers to their respective problems.

Finally, to recap, people have a right to have all the information and not just the information coming from those with a vested interest in keeping the public in the dark. Therefore, it is essential that everyone has all the information about:

- The known risks of the drugs and/or treatment from unbiased, non-conflicted medical review.
- The medical validity of the diagnosis for which drugs are being prescribed.
- All available non-drug options.
- The right to refuse any treatment they consider harmful.

* * *

Chakras

My research into suicide looked at some of the reasons why people take their own lives and introduced me to the concept of chakras. It is believed that at the core of suicide lies a grievance the person holds onto about someone or something. Suicide is basically retaliation. Therefore, one could surmise that taking mind-altering medication may speed up, cause or aggravate people leaning towards this disposition, based on the high number of people who commit suicide whilst taking antidepressants. Suicide ultimately culminates in a separation between mind and body. This *separation* led me to explore in greater detail the meaning of chakras.

Chakra, based on Hindu and Buddhist beliefs, are believed to be centres of the body from which a person can collect energy. The chakras are thought to vitalise the physical body and to be associated with interactions of a physical, emotional and mental nature. The function of the chakras is to attract energy to keep the spiritual, mental, emotional and physical health of the body in balance. They are said by some to unify the soul's earthly journey to connect to the higher power of God.

The Chakra System consists of seven energy points found within the body. Here you find the blueprint for the entire body – mind, body and spirit. All of the charkas are interwoven with each other. The chakras of suicidal people will be completely out of sync, forcing the person to consider that the only solution to release them from their emotional pain is suicide.

The first chakra is located at the base of the spine. It relates to existence. This is the centre of our survival and physical identity.

The second chakra is located below the navel. It relates to our thoughts. This is the centre of our feelings and emotional intelligence.

The third chakra is located in the solar plexus. It relates to ability. This is the centre of our individual identity: ego, willpower, impulses, anger and strength.

The fourth chakra is located in the middle of the chest behind the breast bone (sometimes referred to as the heart chakra). It relates to love. This is the centre of our acceptance of others, and ourselves – of love, forgiveness and compassion.

The fifth chakra is located in the throat. It relates to communication. This is the centre of our internal speech within the mind – how we speak to ourselves – and our ability to hear other people correctly, as well as encompassing our creativity.

The sixth chakra is located in the centre of the forehead (also referred to as the third eye). It relates to intuition – gut instinct. This is the centre of our insight, visualisation and imagination.

The seventh chakra is located in the crown of the head. It relates to knowledge. This is the centre of our belief system, wisdom, spiritual understanding, and our connection/relationship with God or the Higher Spirit.

Recommended treatment

Reiki, first developed by Mikao Usui, a Japanese Buddhist in 1922, is a hands-on healing treatment. It helps cleanse the chakras and unblocks any imbalances in the energetic shallows of the auric system. It repairs the aura, the energetic pathways connected to the body and each individual chakra. The sense of wellbeing felt after a few treatments is believed to be utterly phenomenal.

A paradoxical effect is when medical treatment, usually a drug, has the opposite effect to that which would normally be expected.

Homeopathy and Other Non-Drug Treatments

Homeopathy is a scientific method of treatment, which was developed by the German physician Dr Samuel Hahnemann in the late eighteenth century and is used throughout the world. In India, two-thirds of the population are treated with homeopathic treatments in favour of orthodox medicine. Mahatma Gandhi once said "Homeopathy cures a greater percentage of cases more than any other method of treatment." In Europe, it has also started to become widely recognised and used. Although the principle of homeopathy has been around for several centuries, Hahnemann's work and teachings on the subject are recognised as how homeopathy is known today. In his experiments with natural herbs and plants lay the belief that symptoms of various medical ailments could be produced when tested on healthy individuals but cured when given to people who had become ill naturally – giving credit to his theory that 'like treats like'.

Homeopathy physicians believe that omega-3 fats, which cannot be produced by the human body, are particularly beneficial to its treatment. Studies by Stoll et al. (1999), Su et al. (2003), Davidson et al. (2011), and Krawczyk and Rybakowski (2012) have all shown that people who were deficient in omega-3 fats have enjoyed good results, particularly for those enduring severe depressive episodes, after having taken homeopathic treatment specifically intended to address this deficiency.

Gaier (2011) consolidated the results in these studies by his use of purslane – an edible plant – which he has used to effectively treat bipolar. Purslane can be made into a soup, stir-fried, pureed or mixed into a salad (say, alongside lettuce and avocado pear), or just treated as most other vegetables: Gaier says it has a slightly sour/salty taste but that he has found that even children will learn to eat it. Gaier also acknowledges homeopaths recognition that for the first 250,000 years of humankind, people settled near water and enjoyed a diet of freshly caught fish but over the course of the last 9,000 years man has switched to a grain-based diet and now consumes very little fish oil, which is a major source of omega-3 fats. We are now mainly meat eaters – not fish eaters. Behind this is the belief that *Homo Sapiens*, the modern species of human to which we all belong, have constitutions that still require a regular supply of fish oil, which lies in our DNA and which keeps us healthy both mentally and physically.

"The term 'homeopathy' comes from the Greek words 'homoeos' (meaning 'similar') and 'pathos' (meaning 'suffering'). The principle of homeopathy lies in the Greek philosophy that 'like cures like', i.e. treating an illness with a substance that produces symptoms similar to those from which the person suffers. In other words, a substance which can produce symptoms of disease in a healthy person can remove similar symptoms from the sick when given in homeopathic doses. For example, if you're chopping onions, your eyes water, itch and burn and you may also develop a runny nose with sneezing. If you had this similar pattern of symptoms during a cold or hay fever, then a homeopathic remedy made from red onion (Allium cepa) might be an effective treatment for this condition. Another example would be the use of the homeopathic remedy prepared from coffee, which is often used to treat the same type of insomnia that too much coffee can cause.

Based on the principle of 'like cures like', homeopathy is applicable in the treatment of many acute and chronic conditions. The main goal of a homeopath is therefore to identify the one substance that would produce symptoms most similar to those from which a patient is suffering.

Homeopathic remedies are made from naturally occurring substances, such as plants and minerals. There are thousands of commonly-used remedies and each homeopathic remedy can be used to treat a specific set of symptoms. Rather than giving the same medicine to each patient with the same diagnosis, homeopathic remedies are selected for each person based on the entire symptom picture, in addition to the diagnosis and disease pathology.

How does homeopathy work? To answer this question, one must first understand the basic causes of disease. Disease is a state of imbalance resulting from several factors. These factors include external influences such as lifestyle (diet, exercise), environmental exposures, microbes, as well as physical and mental trauma. However, in order for these external factors to cause a disease, the individual must possess the susceptibility – his/her vitality must be weakened. Vitality is synonymous with energy – the more energetic one feels, the greater the vitality is. If you feel mentally alert and are physically active, you have a strong vital force. If you are vitally strong then you are less susceptible to disease forces. You are more immune to the actions of viruses, bacteria, parasites, seasonal changes and stress – you fall ill less often.

According to the homeopathic way of thinking, a disease originates from the disturbance of this 'vital force' that sustains life, which can be considered as the 'engine' of a person, the physical or mental vigour, the capacity to live. As the origin of the disease occurs on an energetic level it needs an energetic therapy, such as homeopathy, to meet this level. There are other energetic therapies such as herbal medicine or acupuncture, but homeopathy is usually the preferred first choice. The vital force is also influenced by the food one eats, the exercise one takes, medications, and the function of organs, environmental factors and stress. A happy person who loves life, who contributes positively to life and who has aims in life, supports this vital force.

When seeing a homeopath with regards to bipolar depression, the practitioner will first establish if there is an underlying problem with a thyroid disorder or hormonal imbalances and correct them if needed. A homeopath will then establish all the physical and mental symptoms and prescribe the one remedy specific to this person.

The problem most homeopaths face that in the current drug-dependent world, it is not easy to evaluate what the natural 'disease' is, because the drugs will produce a plethora of side-effects and illnesses that are not naturally indicative of the person's wellbeing. In other words, were they not taking psychotropic drugs, they would not have such blurred symptoms – as well as fragile and mental countenance as their presentation. The reality is these artificially induced illnesses (side-effects) are superimposed on the original natural illness, therefore symptoms are contaminated or suppressed and the patient cannot give a clear picture of how they are feeling. Patients under medical supervision should be fifty per cent weaned off psychotropic drugs before homeopathic remedies are given. However, a small amount of homeopathic *organopathic* medicine can be given to assist the withdrawal process and prevent suppressive symptoms that may arise as a result.

There are numerous homeopathic remedies that can be used to treat for bipolar depression as outlined in studies by Adler et al. (2011), Bawden (2012) and Longacre et al. (2012). These remedies come in several forms, including liquid potencies but are usually small pills, which are absorbed under the tongue. It is the skilled homeopath who will prescribe the right medicine in the correct strength to grow the vitality of a patient, which then balances organ functions. In other words: the homeopathic remedy gives the energetic impulse to the body to heal itself and to bring it back into harmony. A homeopath does not treat symptoms but the vital force of the person. Once the patient is back in harmony no further treatment is needed. A homeopath will also give advice on maintaining a balanced lifestyle – and will sometimes direct the patient to see a nutritionist about nutrition and food supplements, as well as naturopathy and herbal medicine, if this is deemed appropriate.

Finally, a person's environment is important for their wellbeing. If a patient is in contact with someone in the family or at work who undermines them by constant criticism, then the patient won't get well. This is something a good homeopath will seek to resolve. It often helps in such cases for the patient to have a word with the other party to address the conflict. Sometimes, if the situation does not improve, a homeopath may recommend a change in living arrangements or job, knowing that a harmonious environment is the best basis on which to get well and stay healthy.

Naturopathy

Naturopathy is an eclectic system of healthcare, which promotes the body's self-healing mechanism. It is in tandem with homeopathy in the sense that it too believes in viewing and treating the whole person and was first used by the Hippocratic School of Medicine in about 400 B.C. Naturopathy aims at finding a cause of disease, and using the laws of nature to induce cure. Its principle believes that the body has a capacity to heal itself because it has its own innate intelligence to do so. Naturopathy assists this process with homoeopathy, acupuncture and herbal medicine.

A naturopath will carry out a lengthy interview with the patient focusing on lifestyle, medical history, emotional tone, and physical features, as well as physical examination which may include a recommendation for pathology testing such as hair, stool, or blood analysis. They will then work with the patient to develop ways at reducing stress, encourage a healthy diet that avoids overeating, tea, coffee, and alcohol along with a lifestyle that includes exercise, as well as the minimisation of pharmaceutical drugs. The treatment plan will also invariably include herbal medicine, homeopathic treatments, or other suitable remedies.

It is estimated that three quarters of lifetime psychiatric disorders start in adolescence, as discovered in a two year study carried out by Jacka et al. in 2011. Based on age, socio-economic status, education, and health behaviours, a 'traditional' dietary pattern characterised by vegetables, fruit, meat, and fish, was associated with lower odds for major depression. A 'western' diet of processed or fried foods, refined grains, sugary products, and beer was associated with higher odds for these psychiatric disorders. A healthy diet was defined as one that included fruit and vegetables as 'core food groups' and included both two or more servings of fruit per day and four or more servings of vegetables, as well as total avoidance of processed foods including chips, fried foods, chocolate, sweets, and ice cream. An unhealthy diet was one high in snack and processed foods. But none of this is new information to Naturopathic Medicine who has been saying this for more than a hundred years, as contained in the 1976 book *Not all in the Mind* by the late Dr Richard Mackarness, which is the base for the popular saying 'You are what you eat.'

Orthomolecular medicine

At this point it is worth mentioning orthomolecular medicine – which sits comfortably between homeopathy, naturopathy and the sections that follows on diet and nutrition. Orthomolecular medicine is rarely used in public psychiatric services, although I have found some psychiatrists who use it in their private practice and are willing to prescribe this to new patients with bipolar not already on psychotropic drugs – or prescribe to those already on psychotropic drugs a skilful blend of both.

It was first developed by an American scientist, Linus Pauling, who in 1968 published a research paper entitled *Orthomolecular Psychiatry*, in which he made the claim that for every conventional medical drug that benefits a patient, there are natural substitutes that could achieve the same effect. This was followed by his announcement of the results of his research into mineral deficiencies, which came up with the following conclusions:

- Enzymes are totally necessary for brain function, and mental illness is partly caused by enzyme dysfunction.
- Vitamins might have important biochemical effects in the prevention of associated deficiency diseases.

Pauling's paper proposed the idea of prescribing large amounts of multivitamins to patients with mental illness, including manic depression, which he believed would cure them because once the body returns to a 'natural' state, moods balance out. In plain terms, orthomolecular medicine is a form of complementary and alternative medicine that seeks to maintain health and prevent or treat diseases. Doctors trained in orthomolecular medicine report that mental health problems including bipolar and depression often have a common cause: insufficient nutrients in the brain. Sometimes a simple deficiency of vitamin D causes depression so before any treatment plan is devised for the patient, a whole series of tests are carried out to establish the exact biochemistry levels of each of the following in the body:

- vitamins
- minerals

- proteins
- antioxidants
- amino acids
- digestive enzymes.

The goal of orthomolecular medicine is to restore the body's optimal state by correcting imbalances, once the levels of deficiency are established.

Each patient will be given a carefully devised treatment plan and dietary advice outlining the relevant vitamins, minerals, trace elements and amino acids, that are needed, aimed at successfully restoring what is lacking in the person's equilibrium. Nutritional supplements may also be prescribed which can be taken along with regular food.

This article was written in close consultation with Dr V. Shah, Dr H. Keppler and Dr. H.C. Gaier who are all leading experts in the field of Homeopathy and Naturopathy. Permission has been granted to reproduce extracts from their works.

The piece on Orthomolecular Medicine was completed after discussion with Dr P.E. Idahosa, a psychiatrist who prescribes this in his private practice.

Gut and Psychology Syndrome (GAPS)

GAPS is an acronym for Gut And Psychology Syndrome, based on the work of Dr Natasha Campbell-McBride. Her research has shown that patients with psychiatric disorders also have digestive problems. Hippocrates, the father of modern medicine, once said, "All disease begins in the gut." Whilst not all individuals with gut dysbiosis experience psychological or psychiatric diseases, its strong presence in psychiatric patients stands out from the patients Dr Campbell-McBride has treated in her clinic.

Psychiatry has created different diagnostic boxes for people, but the reality is that a modern patient does not fit into any of them neatly. Most of us all fit into a lumpy picture of overlapping neurological and psychiatric disorders. When examined in a clinical setting, Dr Campbell-McBride found that apart from so-called mental problems, these people were also physically ill with digestive problems, malnourishment, allergies, asthma, eczema, cystitis and fussy eating patterns.

In her clinic, Dr Campbell-McBride examines the health of each patient – firstly by taking a full account of his/her parents' health history. It is considered that mothers in particularly pass onto their children their unique gut micro-flora at birth. Almost 100% of mothers of children with learning disabilities and mental problems have abnormal gut flora, which they pass to their child. What can damage gut flora? It is a well-known fact that antibiotics have a serious damaging effect on the gut flora, as they wipe out most bacteria, good and bad, leaving room on the mucosal lining of the gastrointestinal tract for opportunistic diseases to grow. Others factors apart from genetics include contraceptive pills which affect the gut, hectic, stressful lifestyles consisting of high stress and anxiety levels, modern diets consisting of fast and processed food along with sugar, coke and low fat diets. The end result is an imbalance of good flora in the gut. When the gut flora is abnormal, the gut becomes a major source of toxicity in the body (instead of being a source of nourishment); large amounts of very toxic chemicals are absorbed into the bloodstream and are carried into the brain, impairing its function. As a result, psychiatric disorders develop, because of the poor health of the gut. The brain is a physical organ: it is a very hungry organ that constantly needs feeding. An unhealthy gut cannot supply necessary nutrients to feed the brain. When a digestive system is full of toxicity, the poison in the gut will get into the brain – hence the manifestation of a psychiatric order like bipolar. GAPS Nutritional Programme is the treatment protocol for this condition. When you get to the root of the problem by finding the underlying cause, then with the help of a certified GAPS Practitioner (you can find one on **www.gaps.me**), healing will take place and recovery is within one to two years.

A full medical examination – including blood and stool testing takes place to check the health of the gut and determine the necessary amount of natural flora for good health is present. A breached gut wall barrier leaves people vulnerable to pathogenic invaders and bacteria that are simply looking for a home.

The majority of people with psychiatric conditions are pale and pasty. When tested, they show various stages of anaemia. To have healthy blood we require many different nutrients and vitamins – B1, B2, B3, and B6, B12, K and D. Minerals lacking include iron, calcium, magnesium, zinc, cobalt, selenium and boron as well as essential amino acids and fats.

GAPS diet

This consists of a diet including meats, fish, eggs, fermented dairy and vegetables (some well-cooked, some fermented and some raw). There is emphasis on homemade meat and fish stock to provide building blocks for the rapidly growing cells of the gut lining as they have a soothing effect on any areas of inflammation in the gut.

Best foods suggested by GAPS:

- eggs
- fresh meat (liver and other organ meats should be eaten on a regular basis)
- fish – fresh or frozen (not smoked)
- shellfish
- fresh vegetables and fruit
- nuts and seeds
- garlic and olive oil.

Probiotic foods:

- plain yoghurt (fruit should not be mixed with dairy)
- kefir
- sauerkraut
- home-made pickle.

Provides information on food to avoid:

- all grains
- sugar
- potatoes (and sweet potatoes)
- parsnips
- yams
- all processed foods.

GAPS practitioners are all over the world, and several clinics in the UK and Ireland will devise personalised diets for their patients. This will include key recommendations for breakfast, lunch and dinner. A GAPS diet is not expensive. All meals are home-made and only fresh, natural ingredients are allowed. Some work and preparation is required but it is not hard work. It is a very wholesome and healthy diet that will allow the person to heal and seal the gut lining and lay a strong foundation for good health for the rest of his or her life.

GAPS can help everyone. Nobody is beyond help. Everyone can be healed. But with psychiatric patients, including those who are diagnosed with bipolar, they are 'drug addicts' in the sense that they are addicted to antidepressants, antipsychotics and mood stabilising medications – all of which they need weaning off over a period of time but under supervised medical care – as given by a GAPS practitioner.

Dr Campbell-McBride's book Gut and Psychology Syndrome outlines in great detail her theories, research and findings linking psychiatric disorders to problems that stem from the gut. Her book contains recipes and suggestions for developing optimum health – but most crucially the ability of GAPS to cure the underlying problem.

Diet and Nutrition

When faced with someone in mental turmoil, doctors so often forget they are physicians. The word physician comes from the Greek word 'phusos', which means nature. In a way it is not the fault of the doctors because they receive twenty minutes, if that, of training in nutrition. The role of nutrition in health is downgraded by being relegated to a supplementary profession, that of dietetics, whereas in fact it is the key factor.

Foods high in sugar and carbohydrates, fatty foods and sugar substitutes, along with caffeine, additives and preservatives, can adversely affect mood and behaviour. Food today is much more devoid of vitamins and minerals than it used to be – particularly nutritional levels of vitamins C, E, A and B along with zinc, magnesium, iron, copper and calcium, which are necessary to maintain a balanced diet for adequate physical and mental health.

Fasting

During a fast you are able to recognise the link between body, mind and spirit; 'We are what we eat.' Important is a dynamic balance between internal and external factors and a more holistic approach to illness. Ideally, food should be our only medicine, but nowadays we need some supplements because food is depleted of nutrients: in the same food, there are now fewer nutrients than there were in the past.

It has been found that bipolar patients are deficient in the following:

- vitamin B6
- vitamin B12
- vitamin C
- omega-3
- fatty acids – as well as folic acid.

Most illnesses stem from a lack or deficiency of three essential elements – namely '*nutritional, emotional and physical*', which causes instability and imbalance. In all cases, but especially for the mentally ill, it is critical to reduce the toxic overload we are exposed to or ingest every day, such as the huge amount of harmful chemicals, heavy metals and other poisonous substances that weaken both mind and body. To help combat this daily assault, it is important to understand and introduce 'natural nutritional foods and supplements' into the diet that support stability, aid recovery and improve overall health. The following suggestions are highly recommended for this purpose:

Charcoal powder: s is one of the most vital products everyone should use daily, but especially important for bipolar sufferers and the mentally ill, as it safely removes most of the poisonous toxins contained in prescription medication, water, the air and food. Effective on toxins such as aluminium and other heavy metals in the body which are known to cause memory loss, mood swings, headaches, forgetfulness, muscle pains and respiratory disorders. Charcoal also removes toxins in drinking water such as fluoride (a poisonous industrial waste material now included in our drinking water supply and oral care products such as toothpaste and mouthwash). Simply drinking one teaspoon of charcoal powder mixed in a glass of water daily, (two hours before or after eating, taking medication or supplements), could safely remove the majority of harmful toxins from the body and brain. Charcoal powder is available from GRAMMA'S online www.grammaseshop.com.

Omega oils 3, 6, 9 with vitamin E: are recognised as 'the building blocks of life', essential for growth, organ function and cellular development: particularly beneficial for brain health and regeneration. This is available from GRAMMA'S online www.grammaseshop.com.

Molasses *(from sugar cane)*: contains all the 'natural' vitamins, minerals and trace elements the body needs for daily health maintenance. Just mix one dessertspoon of molasses with one dessertspoon of fresh lemon juice in a cup (topped up with hot water) and drink. Recommended having twice a day or once if you are diabetic. For an extra boost, include one teaspoon of omega oils 3, 6, and 9. Molasses is available from most health stores. For more information on the amazing benefits of molasses, contact GRAMMA'S to receive a product brochure.

Vitamin C: is found in fresh lemons and limes and is best when added to hot water and drunk first thing in the morning (on an empty stomach), or as mentioned above with molasses. Alternatively, take natural vitamin C (1000mg) supplement daily.

Vitamin D: is mainly obtained from the sun. Just fifteen minutes in the sun every day is sufficient. However, as we do not get sufficient sunshine throughout the year in the

UK, you may need to also take natural vitamin D (1000mg) supplement daily.

Unfortunately, due to the EU Food Supplements Directive, many vitamin and mineral supplements and health products on the market (including in health stores) may be tainted with synthetic, GM (genetically modified) or less potent ingredients. To ensure your supplements are derived from pure natural sources, always remember to read the label or contact the manufacturer for confirmation. Recommended: high strength 'natural' Vitamins C and D from www.grammaseshop.com.

A Balanced Diet: should contain plenty of fresh green leafy vegetables and fruits. Avoid junk or processed foods GM, cloned meats and milk, plus other synthetic foods as these also contain harmful chemicals, synthetic ingredients, animal and human DNA or harmful by-products. As the supermarkets are flooded with 'unlabelled' products and produce containing these things, it is best to buy from local farmers' markets where produce is more fresh, wholesome and cost effective. Eat fresh fruit and vegetables, preferably organic, in season and grown locally. Ideally, more than 50% of food intake should be raw. Avoiding trans-fats is also important. Saturated fats are okay in limited amounts but it is better to avoid animal fats other than butter.

Tryptophan is an amino acid antecedent of the much talked-about neurotransmitter, serotonin – but people need adequate levels of B3, B6, folic acid, vitamin C and zinc in order for tryptophan to break down into serotonin. People with alcohol and drug misuse problems will be low in serotonin.

Meals high in tryptophan:

- oat porridge
- soya milk
- fish – salmon and tuna
- turkey and chicken breast
- baked potatoes
- green beans
- lentils
- avocados
- eggs
- green salad

Filtered water: Try and keep away from drinks that don't correctly hydrate the body, especially coffee and alcohol. People who are anxious or stressed tend to lean towards these and as a result, don't drink enough water. This, coupled with smoking will leave the body dehydrated. This alone can cause feelings of depression, along with a racing heart and irritability. However, our drinking water is not as clean as it appears. It too contains harmful toxins and heavy metals, which need to be avoided, removed or reduced. The most used 'water filter' is the jug with a cartridge. However, the most cost effective are the fitted 'water filter installation' systems. Ideally, drink six to eight glasses of filtered water a day.

Dounne Alexander is an author and health campaigner – and also the founder of the Joining Hands in Health campaign; GRAMMA'S (Specialist Herbal Food Manufacturer); and Chair of the Natural World Organization (NWO).

Pioneering British/Caribbean entrepreneur; voted one of the 100 greatest and most influential black people in British history; honoured by the Queen with the MBE for services to the British Food Industry and the recipient of ten National Awards including the 2011 award for Human Rights plus a 2011 award for outstanding contribution to Complementary and Natural Medicine.

Talking Therapies

A traumatic event is a severe emotional shock. This may be caused by experiencing or witnessing violent crime or injury, including domestic violence, childhood abuse and neglect, the death or suicide of a loved one, being involved in a car crash or getting caught up in a natural disaster like an earthquake, tsunami or severe flooding. A house fire, a fall or other type of accident can also cause severe trauma. A traumatic event often constitutes some sort of danger to life, threat of injury or profound sense of loss. Every person will react to trauma in his or her own unique way, but for many this response will include the fear of it happening again which often manifests itself in recurring flashbacks. Traumatic events also often stimulate physical symptoms, such as irritability, jumpiness, or anxiety and sleep problems – along with memory and concentration difficulties.

Counselling helps a person work through his or her feelings and enables them to recognise the early triggers and signs of a potential episode. Counselling may also include advice on a healthy, balanced lifestyle and the avoidance of stress. But good quality counselling isn't just about doling out advice to the person because this would risk dependency, in which case the counsellor just ends up directing the person to constantly do things that they either don't want to do or that they don't understand.

Counselling is about helping the person get to the bottom of their emotional distress, even when the cause isn't obvious. If the person isn't on medication when they first seek help this will be easier than in instances in which the person's mind has been blighted with psychotropic drugs – but even for those taking medication, counselling is still a way forward and a step in the right direction to getting to the root cause of the underlying emotional trauma.

The counsellor must ask the right questions that will enable his or her client to offer the solutions themselves. It is paramount to allow clients to express their reality so that they can discover for themselves what is the problem, rather than having an opinion forced upon them.

The main pitfall in counselling is evaluating the client's consideration of what the problem is, for example by saying:

It's not that......the way you are feeling is because of the relationship you had with your father.........

The client usually is instinctively correct, so whatever they feel is the problem should be fully explored. Deep down, the client will always know what is causing his or her distress, so a good counsellor should let them find it with their help directing them. By all means, the counsellor should prompt if the answers are not forthcoming, but the client should never be put under pressure to come up with an answer. If they are struggling, a counsellor can help by asking probing questions, such as, "Wwhen was the last time you felt alright?"

A good counsellor is basically a good listener who will allow their client to talk about painful, bothersome feelings in an open, safe and non-judgemental manner. They will guide them towards understanding their life and empowering them to move forward and take personal responsibility for how they want to deal with the problem. Standard questions a counsellor may ask their clients in order to get a clearer understanding of them and how the person functions could include:

- How they feel about themselves – how happy they are?
- To what extent do they feel a sense of meaning and purpose in their life?
- Do they feel able to influence things in their own life, local environment or wider society?
- Do they feel they are dealt with fairly – and are they confident that family and friends acknowledge their problems?
- How they function at a personal level?
- How motivated they are?
- How valued do they feel at work?
- To what extent do they feel in control, especially in work or financial terms?
- How they feel in relation to those around them – i.e. social feelings – and how they function in a social context?
- How they relate to others, and how involved they are in social activities such as volunteering, work, hobbies and community groups?
- Do they feel a sense of belonging to a community or place?
- What is their experience of their neighbourhood, friendships and support networks?

I would recommend counselling that is client-centred because this places the need on helping the person to change, rather than dealing only with the immediate presenting problem. When I was studying for my Master's degree in Mental Health Social Work at King's College in London, I trained under a psychotherapist from the Maudsley Hospital. There I learned the importance of listening and examining the *words* clients use when revealing a problem. Part of my training involved recording a session with a client and then playing it back in group supervision. I was often berated for missing the clues clients dropped into the discussion by not asking the client to clarify a particular *word* that would have better revealed what they meant – or better explained why they were having those thoughts.

Some of the people featured in the *Life Stories* of this book mentioned receiving Cognitive Behavioural Therapy (CBT). Whilst this in one sense is a good thing, because CBT raises confidence and gives a boost to the client who is trapped in a pattern of detrimental thoughts, it is, however, non-beneficial in the longer term. It is an inexpensive therapy, not least because it is time-specific and is usually given only for six appointments (usually to patients stabilised by psychotropic medication) and because of this constraint it fails to delve deep enough into the client's background or childhood to pinpoint exactly what is the underlying issue that causes the dysfunction and distress in the person's life.

A counsellor will have the ability to ask discerning questions or indeed question assumptions that the clients have about themselves because although they only deal with the revealed feelings and emotions that the client presents, they also take into account information that may be being concealed, maybe because it is too painful to initially divulge. Clients hold back, but gradually over time they will allow the counsellor into their own intimate 'inner world'. We all have an inner life that is ticking away inside of us, such as Michael described in his *Life Story* – a life that is full of secrets, fears, desires and fantasies. Sometimes we allow people a sneak preview into this world, but good counselling means going a step further and revealing more by being honest with the counsellor – and with yourself.

Physical Exercise

It is often said that exercise and low moods don't like each other but if you bring both together in a head-to-head argument, exercise will win. Any exercise is a bonus but especially at times of low motivation. A brisk walk will arouse your adrenalin making the blood flow by letting more oxygen into the body. Research has shown that walking is the best single activity that leads to energetic feelings and improves cardiovascular fitness. Exercise is one of the best ways of producing endorphins – proteins in your body that promote a feeling of wellbeing. People come up with excuses not to exercise – a bad back, a painful shoulder or weak knees perhaps, but these can easily be remedied by visiting an osteopath or chiropractor who will alleviate the problem. Breaking through the initial barriers of aches and pains and the body's inertia of not doing any exercise opens the door to new possibilities.

It may appear easier said than done to take up exercise when consumed by a lack of motivation. Therefore it is a good idea to invite a friend or family member to join in these activities, making it less of a chore and more enjoyable. Start by going for a walk, allowing fresh air into your lungs every day for fifteen to thirty minutes. This will start you on the road to living a healthier lifestyle. The key is not to over exercise at the beginning which quickly only leads to resentment, but rather to gradually build up your activity levels. Many people with bipolar are heavy smokers, but smoking only adds to an already long list of health concerns. You have got to try to make this list a little shorter, so taking up exercise is a good time to stop.

Starting a fitness regime with a humble walk is, as Catherine said in her *Life Story*, an activity that is free of charge. This is important to consider as many people on low incomes are unlikely to be able to afford an exclusive gym. In addition to walking there are other low-cost or free opportunities for exercise, like running, cycling and even swimming – all of which will add up to improvements in the lungs, heart and vascular system. Along with releasing mood-lifting endorphins, regular exercise can help to stave off the obesity that is a constant unwelcome side-effect of the plethora of medication frequently endured by those with bipolar. The key to success is to find an exercise or sport that you can enjoy doing every day.

These days that doesn't even have to involve leaving the comfort of your own home. Fitness DVDs are plentiful and inexpensive, and will teach many basic stretching exercises that improve fitness. Doing these exercises will help beat depression and, in addition to feeling better, they will also help to boost energy levels, combat boredom and improve self-esteem. Ultimately, once a person starts to feel the benefits of regular exercise they become interested in addressing their diet. Healthy meals, such as a piece of fish, a salad and an apple, will replace fast-foods or microwave foods that are often full of additives.

Yoga is another type of exercise that crops up favourably in research. Utilising a series of strength and breathing techniques, yoga can boost both physical and mental wellbeing. Regular yoga practice has been shown to help combat depression and reduce stress.

If you would like to become more active, don't be afraid to approach your doctor and ask for help. Many surgeries refer people to health and wellbeing programmes specifically designed to help with exercise, fitness and weight management. The sessions are run by a registered dietician and a qualified exercise instructor – and focus on developing key lifestyle skills to successfully manage exercise and weight loss. Even if this option is not available in the area where you live, you should still approach your GP for advice. There will be something that he/she can do – and at the very least, they should offer guidance along with a referral to a dietician.

This was written in consultation with Ross Minter, an ex-professional UK welterweight boxer who is currently a Director of Queensbury Boxing League in Redhill.

Misalignment of the Spine and Bipolar Disorder

Firstly, the ethos of chiropractic, founded by Dr Daniel David Palmer in 1890, is that the body alone can heal itself if it is maintained in its natural state. The functions of the body are monitored by the brain, which stems and branches out through the nervous system, protected by the skull and the vertebra of the spine. The main purpose of the nervous system is to act as a communication relay network between the brain and the entirety of the body.

The efficiency and efficacy of this communication system becomes compromised through bodily injury, especially to the head and back, and subsequent spinal degeneration. Life throws knocks and blows at the body which take their toll and gradually, or suddenly, reduce it from its natural state; thus self-healing becomes unattainable and one becomes reliant on medical intervention for relief. For example, a child learning to ride their bike falls off and hurts their shoulder and mid-back. A spinal vertebrae is displaced during the accident. After a few days the pain of the accident goes away but the displacement remains, resulting in the nerves, previously protected by the damaged bone, becoming pinched, inflamed or otherwise reduced in functionality. One often finds that the organs reliant on these nerves can then suffer malfunction due to the fact that communication with the brain has been interfered with or severed.

Carrying the weight of the head, the first bone of the spine is located under the skull at the base of the brain. It is called the Atlas – aptly named after the Greek god, who, legend has it, was said to have carried the weight of the world on his shoulders. It has the heavy job of the protective channelling of the brain stem into its evolution as the spinal column. The bone itself is shaped like a ring, into which the brain stem tapers. The Atlas bones, along with the next vertebrae down, called the Axis, are endowed with more freedom of motion than the other spinal bones. Combined, they must allow for rotational motion of the head, and thus because of this increased mobility they become more prone to displacement and misalignment. The Atlas is absolutely vital to brain function and body health. Most vertebrae can sustain a fracture without terminal consequence to the patient, whereas a fracture to the Atlas could result in sudden death.

Dr Erin Elster (2004) carried out extensive research in the field of the effects of misalignment of the upper spine, specifically the Atlas bone. Her research documented several cases in which the realignment of the Atlas and other upper cervical bones by a chiropractor has resulted in marked reduction in the number of bipolar episodes and sustained stabilisation in mood for the patient. Noteworthy from her research is that the majority of bipolar cases had a prior certical (upper spine) trauma, as evidenced by the recall of the patient and confirmed through the use of X-ray or laser imaging. Examples of said trauma were accidental blows to the head as a child, car accidents and even a pole vaulting incident. An initial full physical examination, often using X-ray imaging, is standard practice when you visit a chiropractor and it is very common that the cause of the ailment with which the patient is presenting can be traced back to a prior injury or accident to the affected area. The chiropractor then proceeds to get the bones of the injured area back into their native state, and thus allow the restoration of the brain/body communication network: the nervous system.

The Atlas bone and other cervical displacements interfere with brain and spinal cord functions. Symptoms of misalignment range from mood swings and depression to insomnia, dizziness, seizures, headache, migraine, blurred vision, throat infections, sinusitis, and ear/nose/throat issues, to name but a few. In addition to these, Robinson (1998) discovered mood disorders following brain injuries in a study that looked into traumatic brain injury which resulted in psychiatric disorders due to damage to the prefrontal cortex – whilst Marijnissen et al. (2010) looked at elderly people sufferinging manic episodes and considered that the cause was a subdural haematoma due to a head trauma, possibly caused by patients have fallen and injured themselves. Scientific evidence presented by Mahmood (2001) has suggested a relationship between serotonin levels and bipolar disorder yet a cause or causes for fluctuations in this chemical remains unproven. A primary manufacturing site in the body for serotonin is the base of the brain; thus when the Atlas bone is out of place, undue pressure is exerted on this area and nerve function is debilitated. The governing power of the brain is then reduced due to severed communication channels. Thus a corollary is postulated in that serotonin manufacture is decreased. Incidentally, melatonin, a serotonin derivative, is produced by the Pineal gland, located just at the top of the brain stem. This is also affected by a subluxated Atlas, resulting in sleep problems – also common in bipolar patients.

When the Atlas is adjusted by a chiropractor, and the supporting cervical vertebra aligned, the negative symptoms can, by case observation, begin to subside and the patient can experience a return to normality. Treatment may take several months to produce a change and it is important to seek advice from a chiropractor trained and experienced in the upper cervical area as different chiropractors can have different specialities.

In addition to the above, I thoroughly believe that there is an underlying, hitherto undiscovered physical problem or disease, in every bipolar patient. I believe that the discovery of said pain/disease and the treatment of such (which could involve conventional medical treatment such as antibiotics, resetting a broken limb, etc) is the way forward for the alleviation of mental disorders. Drugging or physically removing or electrocuting the brain not only masks the symptoms, leaving the disease to fester but these actions actually harm the patient more, physically and emotionally, as they are inhumane.

This was written in consultation with Zabrina Collins, Managing Director of Abbey Chiropractic and Wellness Centre, Dublin. Zabrina is a passionate opponent of the use of psychotropic drugs.

Aromatherapy

It has been noted by Davis (1998), Andreescu et al. (2008) and Goodman (2010) that people with bipolar often have very heightened senses and have been shown to respond well to complementary therapies like aromatherapy. Therapies of this kind will reduce the need for medication and help counteract its intolerable side-effects.

As with homeopaths, it is important that aromatherapists compile a detailed case history of the client's health. The therapist will need to know about any medication the client is taking or has been prescribed (this also includes vitamins and herbal remedies) and liaise, if necessary, by gaining permission to contact the client's GP or psychiatrist in order to gain more information. As medications for bipolar have such a wide range of unpleasant side-effects, which will, in effect, be the 'presenting condition' seen by the aromatherapist, the treatment will most probably focus on these rather than on the bipolar itself.

Aromatherapy is a wonderful holistic treatment that uses highly aromatic essential oils derived from plants. Usually these essential oils are combined with base oils and used in massage, but they can also be used via oil burners or compresses. The therapist will discuss the best way to incorporate the oils in a treatment. The oils work in three main ways:

- On a pharmacological level, changes occur within the body as the essential oils enter the bloodstream and their aromatic chemicals interact with different hormones and enzymes in the body, and once having entered the bloodstream have the ability to interact with the body's chemistry.
- On a physiological level, the essential oils affect the different systems of the body,e.g. Lavender and Chamomile have a more calming and relaxing effect on the neurological systems, while oils like Peppermint and Rosemary may have a more stimulating affect.
- On a psychological level, the oils can elicit certain emotional responses. How someone responds to a particular aroma is often connected to the individual's associations with the aromas, as well as individual likes and dislikes.

Some of the side-effects of Lithium and other antipsychotics include muscle aches, pains and tremors and – essential oils, used in combination with massage, can be very helpful in alleviating these as well as helping to promote circulation. It's unlikely that a client having a manic episode would want, or be able, to have an aromatherapy massage. However, aromatherapy blends can be made up in advance and used by the client in the bath or shower, in an oil burner or even on a tissue from which they can inhale the scent every so often. If the client is able to, they can also use the oil blend to massage themselves.

Oils that have antidepressant properties:

- Lavender, Clary Sage and Geranium – Petitgrain, Rose, Sandalwood and Ylang Ylang all help to alleviate symptoms of depression. Lavender is also a great remedy for insomnia.
- Jasmine (this is a very heady oil – men may not take to it as much but it can really promote feelings of self-love and acceptance. This oil can also help if the client is suffering from lethargy).
- Neroli (this oil was described to me as an emotional hug – and it is).
- Orange – but this oil is photosensitising (i.e. increases the reaction of skin to sunlight) which is a side-effect of some antipsychotics.
- Citrus, Orange and floral oils are especially reputed to be natural antidepressants. Many of the citrus oils especially have uplifting, feel-good properties – and the floral oils promote feelings of self-love and acceptance (Orange is again photosensitising).
- Bergamot – it is the uplifting qualities of this oil that make it so beneficial for those suffering from depression and lethargy (note this is also photosensitising)
- Lemon and Melissa are emotionally relaxing, and useful in combatting anxiety.
- Rosemary is very stimulating and energising while also helping to promote clearer thinking.

Manic episodes would require oils that would help to soothe, calm, ground and relax the client. Keep in mind that these oils will also affect the body in other ways – so while they can be used to help to promote feelings of calm and wellbeing, oils such as Lavender, Chamomile and Marjoram also have analgesic properties which mean they can help reduce aches and pain. Chamomile and Geranium are also diuretics so they can also be beneficial if fluid retention is an issue.

Oils that have sedative properties:

- Benzoin, Chamomile, Frankincense, Lavender, Marjoram, Melissa, Neroli and Rose.
- Bergamot.
- Clary Sage (this is a lovely oil – it can stop mental chatter and really bring a sense of wellbeing and 'groundedness').
- Ylang Ylang (this is anotherwonderful oil that can promote feelings of wellbeing and self-love).

Stimulating oils:

- Peppermint (small amount). It is known as cephalic oil in that it clears the mind and can leave a person feeling refreshed and energised. It could be helpful for the side-effects of the bipolar medication – such as digestive upsets, muscle pain, dizzy spells, confusion and headaches.
- Lemongrass (this is a skin irritant and skin sensitising oil so more caution is needed if using. It must be diluted more than other oils). This is an uplifting and cheerful oil so it may be more beneficial for when a client is feeling depressed and low. It is best used in a burner as it can be very irritating on the skin – and also can only be used for a few days at a time.

- Balancing and calming oils include:
- Palmarosa has many benefits that can help with some side-effects of medication, but it is also a very good stress-busting oil. It blends beautifully with other oils such as Sandalwood, Orange, Ylang Ylang and Lavender.
- Frankincense is a wonderfully calming oil and it works well on respiratory conditions – it seems to promote slower, deeper and more relaxed breathing, which calms the mind and can help relieve anxiety.
- Cedarwood is an oil that is good for helping to relieve stress and tension.
- Orange and Juniper is a lovely blend – the orange is very uplifting but also sedative while juniper is really an overall tonic for the mind and body. It can help clear mental clutter and promote a refreshed and more positive view of things.
- Jasmine, Neroli and Ylang Ylang are fantastic oils to reduce anxiety and promote self-love and self-acceptance.
- Grapefruit oil helps instil a positive feeling in people. It acts as a mild stimulant that promotes feelings of slight euphoria. Thus you feel uplifted, refreshed and very positive.
- Petitgrain – this is really helpful for people suffering with nervous exhaustion, stress and anxiety. It really works on calming the mind and promoting a general feeling of wellbeing.

This was written in consultation with Meagan Gaskell, who is a qualified aromatherapist, holistic massage therapist and reflexologist. An accident in 1995 helped her realize the importance of good health and that it should not be taken for granted. Through her practice she provides an initial basis of healing while encouraging clients to think and act differently about their lifestyles, promoting in the process better physical and emotional health.

Education, Training and Employment

The importance of learning new skills is that it opens up fresh opportunities and helps deflect attention away from oneself onto new things. There has been ample research done that looks at the link between creativity and bipolar. Collingwood (2010), Figueroa (2005) and Gillett (2005) all examine this link and acknowledge that for people who are diagnosed with bipolar disorder creativity offers a powerful means of expression. Depression in particular is all-consuming – it makes the person internalise too much and externalise too little. In other words, they think too much about themselves and their problems and become shut off from the rest of the world, so the opening up of new avenues of learning is essential to good emotional health and personal growth. The joy of learning something new – that it stimulates thought and opens up new horizons – makes it a viable option in tandem with the other working solutions featured in this part of the book. I feel it is a definite way forward to a new life once a person has sorted out other key areas, for example, medication and stability, diet, exercise, sleep and relaxation, as well as avoiding triggers that cause them stress and anxiety. Learning a new skill is about seeing life from a new perspective – discovering new information, opening up the mind to fresh knowledge and thus increasing self-worth, which can never be achieved by merely taking medication, or indeed by just talking to a therapist about your problems.

Higher education

You will have seen in the Life Stories that some of the contributors have degrees. However, the majority, like so many others with bipolar in mainstream society, will not be so advantaged. Their condition will have greatly interrupted their education and careers – but this can be rectified because there are many routes to take in further and higher education, with many degrees, diplomas and certificate courses available in colleges and universities in the subject area of your choice. There is also the option of home study, with the Open University being a popular choice, although there are several others. The advantage of studying at home is that you have the benefit of doing it at your leisure, although you must be determined to commit to the course. You will have access to a personal tutor, group tutorials and weekend seminars. Most mature students who have been out of education for a while first choose to go on a foundation course that prepares them for the rigours of higher education. This allows them to get into a routine of reading academic text books, writing assignments, meeting deadlines and sitting examinations. However, individuals who are not persuaded to study for a degree might wish to consider vocational courses or apprenticeships in a wide range of subjects. Although these are more practical in nature, they will contain a certain amount of theory and academia.

Employment

Studying is not for everyone and many just want to get a job, although this is not always easy if you have been out of work for some time owing to your bipolar – or you have few qualifications or little work experience. I do know through my experience as a social worker that there are many schemes, training courses and voluntary work opportunities available that prepare people with gaps in their curriculum vitae to re-enter the workforce. I also know that whichever route a person wants to take, the answer is easily accessed on the internet or at your local library, which will be helpful in providing information on courses and opportunities that may not always be well advertised. Likewise, in addition to current job vacancies, your local job centre will direct you to suitable training courses – and to advisors who will help with preparing your curriculum vitae as well as sharing interview techniques.

Leisure courses

Check out prospectuses that are available in your local library, adult education centres and online. Most adult education centres run short-to-medium courses in a range of subjects for several different interest groups across the spectrum of creative skills, health and leisure, self-development, languages and computers – take for example:

- Photography
- Drawing and painting
- Interior design
- Sculpture
- Silversmith/jewellery making
- Cooking
- Music – learn to play an instrument

- Alternative Therapies
- Tai Chi and Yoga
- Massage
- Childcare and Development
- Genealogy
- Creative writing
- Learn a new language – French, German or Spanish etc.
- Computers and Information Technology.

Lying in bed all day and staring at the walls can hardly be therapeutic or beneficial in any way. Rushing around in hyperactivity can hardly be conducive to productivity. As you will have read in the *Life Stories* there is a bohemian, creative side to bipolar that manifests itself more so than with other so-called mental illnesses. You will have seen how creative, intelligent and reflective many of the people are, along with some who have a burning ambition for justice and peace. But somehow years of psychiatric care, years of taking a plethora of various medications with intolerable side-effects, sees the vigour in the person become more and more strained, diminishing the ability for that person to survive, grow and thrive.

Life passes by so quickly and there comes a moment when procrastination becomes embarrassing. You arrive at the 'it's now or never' moment when some action is needed if change is ever going to occur. There is a wealth of new skills to be learned but they, like all the other suggestions in this section, need a modicum of motivation in order to become a reality.

If motivation is difficult, as mentioned earlier, the simplicity of taking a walk and looking at things around you can be very therapeutic – or just finding something to laugh about and forcing yourself to laugh out loud is said to be effective in lifting one's spirits. Whichever works for you will be far more advantageous than being doped up on drugs with your feelings and emotions numbed down.

Afterword

Mary Maddock
Co-Founder of
MindFreedom Ireland

When Declan Henry approached me to write this Afterword for his new book, I was happy to oblige, as I feel it asks important questions of established psychiatry and the need for alternative approaches. When I subsequently discovered that Declan was from a village in Sligo, very close to my own native village of Gurteen, I felt I was helping out a neighbour!

People who have severe mental/emotional/social life problems do not find solutions because:

1. The emphasis in psychiatry is predominately on the coercive, paternalistic, fraudulent, non-scientific medical model. While alternative methods do exist, they are underfunded and outside the mainstream and are almost always dismissed by established psychiatry, very often with the guiding hand of the pharmaceutical industry.

2. Once a person is in need of help, they can be forced into the 'mental health' system and given a non-scientific, discriminatory label and be forcefully treated with toxic drugs which, in the long term, will cause much more harm than good.

3. They will become non-citizens because they will have no legal rights. They will be considered to be brain-

damaged, unable to determine their own lives and in
need of those who 'know best' to act on their behalf.

4. Then they are considered disabled. They will need
maintenance drug treatment for the rest of their
lives, which, in the long term, will only increase and
multiply their original problems.

Since the advent of psychotropic drugs in the 1950s, so-
called mental health problems are increasing at an alarming
rate. Now, because of the amount of fictitious psychiatric
diagnoses, anyone can find himself or herself labelled
'mentally ill'. Living in our increasingly troubled world,
anyone with the 'symptoms' of being human is in danger
of becoming labelled with a psychiatric 'diagnosis'. Then
they can be forced to receive toxic, mind-altering drugs and
electroshock. In Ireland, it is still legal to force psychosurgery
on innocent victims!

I, like so many others, was a victim of fear, force and
fraud at the hands of institutional psychiatry. I encountered
psychiatry for the first time two days after the birth of my
first child. Having received Nitrous Oxide and a neuroleptic
called Sparine in labour, to both of which I was allergic, and
more drugs immediately after the birth, I was whisked off
two days later to a psychiatric hospital where I got my first
electroshock the next day. I subsequently received twelve
more shocks along with multiple sessions of neuroleptic
torture over a six-week period. I often received the
neuroleptics in forced injection form. I can remember the
pain even though, due to the electroshocks and psychotropic
drugs, I would have known very little about it at all, but
managed to acquire my records many years later. All of this

was without consent. I didn't sign any forms and I knew nothing about this medically-induced harm, which was done in the name of 'help'.

I only found out all of this more than three decades after the severe damage and trauma I endured as a first-time mother. I had become a long-term psychiatric slave enduring horrific effects from psychotropic drugs, which I thought was a 'mental illness' I had acquired due to a chemical imbalance in my brain. I thought I had become a different person in need of lifelong 'treatment'.

This is the outrageous fraud and deception most psychiatrists sing from their hymn sheet. This is the reason why so many people like me are being brain-damaged by people who have no cure! When so-called doctors can inflict brain-damage so easily, when they can even do it forcefully, when they are protected legally, when they are aided by governments and insurance companies, it is no wonder that those labelled by psychiatry often live in constant fear. Then fear is the root cause of a troubled mind and a shattered spirit. Is it any surprise that people with real psycho/social difficulties fail miserably to find true peace of mind, body and spirit?

In liberating myself from the clutches of psychiatry, fear was the biggest obstacle I had to overcome. I had been given the manic depressive/bipolar label and one of the three drugs I was prescribed was Lithium. A booklet I was given at the time by the Mood Disorder Fellowship warned that failing to take the Lithium would leave me with a 70% chance of a relapse. I was also scared of ever having to return to hospital after my six previous visits. But the more I educated myself on the toxic effects of the drugs, the more scared I became of the adverse effects of those drugs. A friend of mine was admitted to hospital with severe kidney damage after many years of prescribed Lithium. My own physical health was also deteriorating. My weight had rocketed, I had severe induced Parkinson's, I was losing my hair, my cognitive abilities were seriously impaired and my kidneys too were being affected. Another important factor in my decision to wean myself off the drugs was the strong support of my husband, who promised me he would not send me back to hospital. I also had support from a doctor who was a personal friend and from a second psychiatrist whom I contacted. MindFreedom International provided more support. MFI campaigns for a non-violent revolution of freedom, equality, truth and human rights in the mental health system. The contacts I made through MFI with others who had weaned themselves off their drugs were also hugely important. Three influential books were of further great significance. These were *Toxic Psychiatry* by Dr Peter Breggin, *Beyond Prozac* by Dr Terry Lynch and *Coming off Psychiatric Drugs* by Peter Lehmann. So very gradually I first began to reduce the Largactil over a period of approximately two years and then the Lithium over a further year, doing so all the time under informed supervision. In hindsight I should have taken longer with the Lithium. It wasn't easy. I experienced many withdrawal symptoms including fainting spells, nausea, insomnia and hot flushes. But I persevered and can look back now at the spring of 2000 when I took the last Lithium tablet. The subsequent feeling of liberation and rejuvenation over the past twelve years has been my reward.

*"Of all tyrannies, a tyranny sincerely exercised
for the good of its victims may be the most
oppressive."* C. S. Lewis.

Where there is no choice, there is tyranny. Biopsychiatry offers little or no choice. It only has tunnel vision. It sees people as objects to be fixed, ironically breaking and destroying them in the process. The result is the revolving door syndrome with people being admitted, released and re-admitted to hospital again and again. But in spite of this tyranny, it is encouraging that many people have broken free from the destructive and coercive harm institutional biopsychiatry has left in its wake and have survived and thrived. They are exceptional people. They are today's prophets. They are writers, poets, artists, musicians and true scientists. They are caring, compassionate, empathetic and above all heartfelt people. Their voices must be listened to.

I have recovered/thrived and become a stronger and happier person because I finally found out that many psychiatrists are doctors of deception who destroy people like me. I also found some true doctors such as Dr Terry Lynch, Dr Peter Breggin, Dr Pat Bracken, the late Dr Michael Corry, the late Dr Leon Mosher and the late Dr Thomas Szasz, all of whom bravely challenged the practices of modern psychiatry and found themselves ostracised as a result. Then I became an activist for reform and enlightenment.

I joined MindFreedom International and soon afterwards I helped to co-found MindFreedom Ireland with my husband and lifelong partner Jim. We have written about our relationship with psychiatry in *Soul Survivor – A Personal*

Encounter with Psychiatry, which was first published in 2006. Today I am proud to be a board member of MindFreedom International. I joined other organisations, such as ENUSP (European Network of ex/Users and Survivors of Psychiatry) of which I was a board member and I am a member of INTAR (International Network Towards Alternatives and Recovery).

I discovered mindfulness and practice it daily. This is where I live 'in the moment'. The past has gone and the future has yet to come. I found using my sense of touch in water, combined with my sense of hearing while listening to music, to be the most effective way of achieving mindfulness. Then I could relax and abandon myself to the water while floating with true peace of mind, body and spirit. It has brought me to my senses and I rediscovered my love for music and dancing. Music is indeed our universal emotional language. I, like Abba, say everyday "Thank you for the music."

When mind-altering drug treatment is the first response, people are in danger of becoming lifelong addicts or taking their own lives or the lives of others. On World Suicide Prevention Day, I heard former Irish rugby international Gerry McLoughlin on a radio show speak about his recovery from severe distress because he learned how to practise daily meditation. He did not have recourse to psychotropic drugs.

It is all about choice. If, after being fully informed on all aspects of psychotropic drugs, some people are still content to take that road, so be it. But for people who don't and for people who want to wean themselves off psychotropic drugs, there must be structures put in place to enable them to do so. It can be done. As you will have discovered from this book, there are places where it is being done and people who are willing to help, but government policy needs to invest heavily in the provision of many more such places and alternative practices.

This is the road to true recovery and transformation. This is the road to self-discovery and empowerment. This is the revolution we seek to achieve.

Acknowledgements

I have worked with many people in the writing of this book and therefore need to extend thanks and gratitude to a large number of individuals across a wide spectrum.

Sincere thanks to Lady Margaret McNair and Brian Daniels from the Citizens Commission on Human Rights, who were a supremacy of knowledge. Their vision of a world without psychiatry filled me with inspiration. Special thanks also to Liz Ostermann for her help.

The following professionals provided much valuable assistance to me in sharing knowledge in their respective specialist areas for the book: Professor B.K. Puri, Dr P.E. Idahosa, Dr N. Campbell McBride, Dr V. Shah, Dr H. Keppler and Dr H.C. Gaier, Dounne Alexander, Ross Minter, Meagan Gaskell and Zabrina Collins.

I offer much gratitude to all the kind interviewees featured in *Life Stories* for their time and contribution of their experiences of living with bipolar.

I would like to add a special mention to John Robinson for his poignant poems used in Daniel's story and to Dympna Connaire for the use of her poems in Sean's story.

I thought it was appropriate to choose Mary Maddock from MindFreedom Ireland to write the closing words to the book because I am an ardent admirer of her bravery. Mary was the victim of psychiatric abuse for more than two decades before she realised she was suffering from adverse side-effects to psychotropic medication, as opposed to bipolar, which her psychiatrist has diagnosed. Since withdrawing from the medications, she has been completely well for over a decade.

Much thanks to my publishers at Squirrel Publishing and at York Publishing Services – especially Duncan Beal, Clare Brayshaw and Jo Tozer.

Special recognition and appreciation to Ruth Ryan who designed the captivating sketch for the jacket cover.

I would also like to mention Patricia Hardwicke, my previous editor who worked with me on *Glimpses* and *Buried Deep in my Heart* – who sadly died in the early stages of the book after a long illness. Patricia advised me on an earlier draft of the book, such was her commitment to living as normal a life as possible as her time drew to an end. I paid special thanks and appreciation to her during private prayers at her funeral.

Finally, to the staff at the British Library for their patience and diligence in assisting me with finding the relevant books, journals and articles necessary during the research element of the book. I hope I wasn't too demanding, but I suspect I was at times!

References

Adler, U.C. et al. (2011) Homeopathy for depression. *Trials* 12, 43. doi: 10.1186/1745-6215-12-43.

Andreescu, C. et al. (2008) Complementary and alternative medicine in the treatment of bipolar disorder – a review of the evidence. *Journal of Affective Disorders* 110(1), 16–26.

Bawden, S. (2012) Running an NHS community homeopathy clinic: 10-year anniversary 2001–2011. *Homeopathy* 101(1), 51–56. doi: 10.1016/j.homp.2011.10.003.

Breggin, P. (2012) *Psychiatric drug withdrawal: a guide for prescribers, therapists, patients and families.* Springer Publishing Co Inc.

Collingwood, J. (2010) The link between bipolar disorder and creativity. *Psych Central.*

Darton, K. (2011) *Making sense of antidepressants.* Mind booklet.

Davidson, J.R. et al. (2011) Homeopathic treatments in psychiatry: a systematic review of randomized placebo-controlled studies. *Journal of Clinical Psychiatry* 72(6), 795–805. doi: 10.4088/JCP.10r06580.

Davis, P. (1998) Aromatherapy: an A–Z. CW Daniel Company Ltd, UK; revised edition.

Diagnostic and Statistical Manual of Mental Disorders 5 (2013) American Psychiatric Association; 5th edition.

Elster, L. (2004) Treatment of bipolar, seizure and sleep disorders and migraine headaches utilizing a chiropractic technique. *Journal of Manipulative and Physiologic Therapeutics* 27(3), 217. doi: 10.1016/j.jmpt.2003.12.027.

Figueroa, C.G. (2005) Virginia Woolf as an example of a mental disorder and artistic creativity. *Revista Medica de Chile* 133, 1381–88.

Fras, I. et al. (1967) Comparison of psychiatric symptoms in carcinoma of the pancreas with those in some other intra-abdominal neoplasms. *American Journal of Psychiatry*, 123(12), 1553–1562.

Gaier, H.C. (2011) Anthropology holds clues to what is 'natural'. *British Naturopathic Journal* 28(2): 8–10.

Gillett, G. (2005) The unwitting sacrifice problem. *The Journal of Medical Ethics* 31, 327–332.

Glenmullen, J. (2006) *Coming off antidepressants.* Constable and Robinson Ltd.

Goodman, S. (2010) *Bipolar: special aromatherapy blends for difficult times.* Natural Healistic Website.

Hall, R.C.W. et al. (1978) Physical illness presenting as psychiatric disease. *Archives of General Psychiatry* 35, 1315–1320.

Healy, D. (2004) *Psychiatric drugs explained.* Churchill Livingstone; 4th edition.

International Classification of Diseases (1992) World Health Organization.

Krawczyk, K. and Rybakowski, J. (2012) Augmentation of antidepressants with unsaturated fatty acids omega-3 in drug-resistant depression. *Psyciatria Polska* 46(4), 585–98 (in Polish).

Longacre, M. et al. (2012) Complementary and alternative medicine in the treatment of refugees and survivors of torture: a review and proposal for action. *Torture* 22(1), 38–57.

Mahmood, T. (2001) Serotonin and bipolar disorder. *Journal of Affective Disorders* 66(1), 1–11.

Marijnissen, R.M. et al. (2010) First manic episode in the elderly – consider a subdural haematoma due to head trauma as cause. *Cerebrovascular Diseases* 31(1) 154, A1235 (in Dutch).

McKeon, P. (1997) *Bipolar disorder: a practical guide book.* Aware, Ireland.

Mental Health Act, The (1983) Department of Health, UK.

Moore, T.J. (1998) *Prescription for disaster.* Simon and Schuster.

Pauling, L. (1968). Orthomolecular psychiatry. Varying the concentrations of substances normally present in the human body may control mental disease. *Science* 160(3825), 265–271.

Petry, N.M. et al. (2008) Overweight and obesity are associated with psychiatric disorders. *Psychosomatic Medicine* 70, 288–297.

Raphael, D. (2009) Restructuring society in the service of mental health promotion: are we willing to address the social determinants of mental health? *International Journal of Mental Health Promotion* 11(3), 18–31.

Robinson, R.G. et al. (1998) Comparison of mania and depression after brain injury: causal factors. *American Journal of Psychiatry* 145, 172–178.

Soreff, S. et al. (2002) Bipolar affective disorder. *eMedicine Journal* 3(1).

Sternberg, D.E. (1986) Testing for physical illness in psychiatric patients. *Journal of Clinical Psychiatry* 47(1), 5.

Stoll, A.L. et al. (1999) Omega-3 fatty acids in bipolar disorder: a preliminary double-blind, placebo-controlled trial. *Archives of General Psychiatry* 56, 407–412.

Su, K.P. et al. (2003) Omega-3 fatty acids in major depressive disorder: a double-blind, placebo-controlled trial. *European Neuropsychopharmacology* 13, 267–271.

Tubridy, A. and Corry, M. (2001) *Depression: an emotion not a disease*. Mercier Press.

Vieta, E. and Phillips, M.L. (2007) Deconstructing bipolar disorder: a critical review of its diagnostic validity and a proposal for DSM-V and ICD-11. *Schizophrenia Bulletin* 33(4), 886–892.

Webster, R. (1995) *Why Freud was wrong (sin, science and psychoanalysis)*. Orwell Press.

Bibliography

Adams, M. (2007) Natural *Health Solutions*. Truthpublishing

Alexander, D. (2001*) A Mission of Love*. Unity Books Ltd

Andre, L. (2009) *Doctors of Deception*. Rutgers University Press

Angell, M. (2005) *The Truth about the Drug Companies: How They Deceive Us and What to Do about It*. Random House Trade; Reprint edition

Bassman, R. (2007) *A Flight to Be*. Tantamount Press

Bentall, R.P. (2010) *Doctoring the Mind: Why psychiatric treatments fail*. Penguin

Blake –Tracy, A. (1994) *Prozac Panacea or Pandora*. Cassia Publications

Breggin, P. (2007) *Your Drug May Be Your Problem: How and Why to Stop Taking Psychiatric Medications*. Da Capo Press Inc; Revised edition

Brondolo et al (2008) *Break the Bipolar Cycle: A Day by Day Guide to Living with Bipolar Disorder: A Day to Day Guide to Living with Bipolar Disorder*. McGraw-Hill Contemporary

Breggin, P. (2009) Medication Madness: The Role of Psychiatric Drugs in Cases of Violence, Suicide, and Crime. St. Martin's Griffin

Breggin, P. (2009) *Medication Madness: The Role of Psychiatric Drugs in Cases of Violence, Suicide, and Crime.* St. Martin's Griffin. Reprint edition

Breggin, P. (2010) *Toxic Psychiatry: Why Therapy, Empathy and Love Must Replace the Drugs, Electroshock and Biochemical Theories of the New Psychiatry.* Flamingo; (Reissue) edition

Burton, N. (2009) *Living with Bipolar Disorder.* Sheldon Press

Campbell-McBride, N. (2010) *Gut and Psychology Syndrome.* Medinform Publishing; 2nd Revised edition

Caplan. P.J (1995) *They Say You're Crazy.* Addison Wesley Publishing Company

Carlat, D. (2010) *Unhinged: The Trouble with Psychiatry – A Doctor's Revelations about a Profession in Crisis.* Free Press: First edition

Carter, J.P. (1998) *Racketeering in Medicine: The Suppression of Alternatives.* Hampton Roads Publishing Co. First Printing edition

Corry, M. and Tubridy, A. (2001) Going *Mad?: Understanding Mental Illness* Newleaf

Evans et al (2011) *Testing Treatments: Better Research for Better Healthcare.* Pinter & Martin Ltd. 2nd edition

Goldacre, B. (2009) *Bad Science.* Harper Perennial

Goldacre, B. (2012) Bad *Pharma: How drug companies mislead doctors and harm patients.* Fourth Estate

Greenberg, G. (2010) *Manufacturing Depression: The Secret History of a Modern Disease* Bloomsbury Publishing PLC

Healy, D. (2006) *Let Them Eat Prozac: The Unhealthy Relationship Between the Pharmaceutical Industry and Depression (Medicine, Culture, and History).* New York University Press: New edition

James, A. (2001) *Raising our Voices.* Handsell Publishing

Johnson, B. (2006) *Unsafe at any dose.* Trust Consent Publishing

Johnstone, L. (2000) Users and Abusers of Psychiatry: A Critical Look at Psychiatric Practice. Routledge; 2nd edition

Jones et al (2009) *Coping with Bipolar Disorder: A CBT-Informed Guide to Living with Manic Depression.* Oneworld Publications

Kent, T.K. (2012) *Lectures on Homeopathic Philosophy.* Lightning Source UK Ltd

Kirsch (2009) *The Emperor's New Drugs: Exploding the Antidepressant Myth.* Bodley Head

Kutchins, H (1999) *Making Us Crazy: DSM – The Psychiatric Bible and the Creation of Mental Disorders.* Constable

Law, J. (2006) *Big Pharma: How the world's biggest drug companies market illness.* Robinson Publishing

Laing, R. (2010) *The Divided Self: An Existential Study in Sanity and Madness.* Penguin Classics

Last, C.G. (2009) *When Someone You Love is Bipolar: Help and Support for You and Your Partner.* Guilford Press

Lehmann, P. (1998) *Coming Off Psychiatric Drugs.* Peter Lehmann Publishing

Lynch, T. *Beyond Prozac.* Marins Books

Mackarness, R. (1976) *Not all in the Mind*

Maddock, M. (2006) Soul Survivor – *A Personal Encounter With Psychiatry.* Asylum Publishers

Martensson, L. (1998) *Deprived of our Humanity.* The Voiceless Movement

McManamy, J. (2006) *Living Well with Depression and Bipolar Disorder: What Your Doctor Doesn't Tell You That You Need to Know.* HarperCollins

Medawar et al (2004) *Medicines Out of Control?* Aksant Academic Publishers

Moncrieff, J. (2009) *A Straight Talking Introduction to Psychiatric Drugs (Straight Talking)*. PCCS Books

Moncrieff, J. (2009) *The Myth of the Chemical Cure: A Critique of Psychiatric Drug Treatment*. Palgrave Macmillan; Revised edition

Mosher, L.R. (2004) *Soteria: Through Madness to Deliverance*. Xlibris Corporation

Null et al (2011) *Death by Medicine*. Praktikos Press

O'Meara (2006) *Psyched Out*. AuthorHouse

Owen et al (2007) *Bipolar Disorder – The Ultimate Guide*. Oneworld Publications

Puri, B. (2005) *The Natural Way to Beat Depression: The Groundbreaking Discovery of EPA to Successfully Conquer Depression*. Hodder Paperbacks; New edition

Rapley et al (2011) *De-Medicalizing Misery: Psychiatry, Psychology and the Human Condition*. Palgrave Macmillan

Redfield Jamison, K. (2011) *An Unquiet Mind: A memoir of moods and madness*. Picador

Roberts (2011) *Bipolar Disorder: The Essential Guide*. Need-2-Know

Rowe, D. (1987) *Beyond Fear*. Fontana

Sanders, P. (2003) *The Tribes of the Person-Centred Nation: an introduction to the schools of therapy related to the person-centered approach.* PCCS Books. 2nd edition

Stastny, P. et al (2007) *Alternatives Beyond Psychiatry*. Peter Lehmann Publishing

Szasz, T. (1977) *The Manufacture of Madness*. Harper and Row, Publishers

Szasz, T. (1987) *Insanity the idea and its consequences*. John Wiley and Sons, Inc

Szasz, T.S. (2007) *The Medicalization of Everyday Life: Selected Essays*. Syracuse University Press

Szasz, T.S. (2008) *Psychiatry: The Science of Lies*. Syracuse University Press

Szasz, T.S. (2010) *The Myth of Mental Illness*. HarperCollins; Revised edition

Szasz, T.S. (2011) *Suicide Prohibition: The Shame of Medicine*. Syracuse University Press

Timimi, S. (2009) *A Straight-talking Introduction to Children's Mental Health Problems (Straight Talking Introductions)* PCCS Books

Walker, M.J. (2011) *Dirty Medicine – The Handbook*. Slingshot Publications; First edition

Watters, E. (2011) *Crazy Like Us: The Globalization of the Western Mind.* Robinson Publishing

Whitaker, R. (2010) *Anatomy of an Epidemic: Magic Bullets, Psychiatric Drugs, and the Astonishing Rise of Mental Illness in America.* Crown Publishing Group

Whitaker, R. (2010) *Mad in America: Bad Science, Bad Medicine, and the Enduring Mistreatment of the Mentally Ill.* Basic Books; 2nd edition

Index